THE OFFICIAL
M.D.
HANDBOOK

THE OFFICIAL M.D. HANDBOOK

By Anne Eva Ricks, M.D.

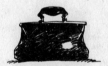

Artwork by Jon McIntosh

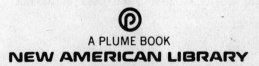

A PLUME BOOK
NEW AMERICAN LIBRARY
TIMES MIRROR
NEW YORK AND SCARBOROUGH, ONTARIO

Copyright © 1983 by Anne Eva Ricks

Artwork Copyright © 1983 by Jon McIntosh

Photography by Chas. E. Martin

 PLUME TRADEMARK REG. U.S. PAT. OFF. AND FOREIGN COUNTRIES
REGISTERED TRADEMARK—MARCA REGISTRADA
HECHO EN HARRISONBURG, VA., U.S.A.

SIGNET, SIGNET CLASSIC, MENTOR, PLUME, MERIDIAN AND NAL BOOKS
are published *in the United States* by The New American Library, Inc.,
1633 Broadway, New York, New York 10019, *in Canada* by The New
American Library of Canada Limited, 81 Mack Avenue, Scarborough,
Ontario M1L 1M8

Library of Congress Cataloging in Publication Data

Ricks, Anne Eva.
   The official M.D. handbook.

   1. Medicine—Vocational guidance—Anecdotes, facetiae, satire,
etc. 2. Medicine—Vocational guidance—Miscellanea. I. McIntosh,
Jon. II. Title. III. Title: Official MD handbook. [DNLM: 1. Students,
Medical—Popular works. 2. Physicians—Popular works. W 21 R5390]
R690.R5   1983   610'.207   83-8336
ISBN 0-452-25438-8

First Printing, October, 1983

1 2 3 4 5 6 7 8 9

PRINTED IN THE UNITED STATES OF AMERICA

For Elliott

Acknowledgments

Many thanks to Mom and Dad, who shelled out for four years of sustained foolishness, and to my far-flung sibs Dave, Lynn, Peg, Mike, Rick, Mary Catherine, and Sarah. Special thanks to Tom, who suggested I quit talking and write a book. The editing by members of the Russell clan at Thanksgiving was remarkable for its excellence as well as tact. I am indebted to Dr. Arden Wander, the brilliant cornea-transplant specialist, for being my mentor (whether he wanted to or not).

I am grateful to my colleagues, who risked everything from broken engagements to dismissal from residency for posing in these photographs—I hope your patients never see them!—Dr. Nancy Bagamery, Dr. Terry Baird, Dr. William Boozan, Dr. Jefferson Burroughs, Dr. Allan Chamberlain, Dr. Christopher Conner, Dr. Sharron Dupler, Dr. Theodore Fifer, Dr. Mary Gaskill, Dr. Mindy Hastie, Dr. Jonathan Lease, Dr. Nancy Loy, Dr. Maury Luxembourg, Dr. Jack Leibold, Dr. Becky Mortenson, Dr. Jeffrey Mueller, Dr. Jeffrey Nudleman, Dr. Deanna Parobeck, Donald Ott, Dr. Joseph Ross, Dr. James Schmidt, Dr. Elliott Sumers, Dr. Robert Thomas, Dr. Barbara Wilson, and Dr. Patti Young. Special thanks to Dr. Melisa Rizer, whose home phone will henceforth be unlisted. May Hippocrates forgive you all.

This book would not have been delivered without the obstetrical talents of my encouraging ("Push! Push!") editor, Ann Waterfall, and my optimistic ("*Sure* there's a book in there!") agent, Donald Cutler. Bookbirthing is an overrated experience, though. Next time I'll skip the Lamaze and go for a saddle block.

Contents

4: So What's Medical School Really Like? or, In the Fundus of the Beast 19

5: Strangers in a Strange Land: Medical Students on the Hospital Wards 27

6: The Doctor's Social Life, and Other Overrated Phenomena 33

7: Choosing A Specialty 62

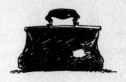

9: Looking for a Residency in All the Wrong Places 99

8: Specialists: An Inside Look 83

10: The Intern's Survival Manual for Guerrilla Warfare 105

11: Private Practice
112

12: Patients:
A Field Guide
to Wild Species   130

13: Those Strangers
to Whom You've
Dedicated Your Life:
Your Patients   133

14: Customer
Relations; or, Coping
(Professionally) with
Your Patients   141

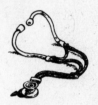

CHAPTER 1

You, Too, Can Be a Doctor

Remember the last time you visited the doctor?

You told him about your troublesome sinuses; he gave you a perfunctory look-over, handed you a prescription for five dollars' worth of antibiotic, and charged you seventy-five dollars?

Did it occur to you then, "Hey, *I* could be a doctor!"

Or how about the last time you were chatting it up in the local singles bar with a good-looking member of the opposite sex, when a doctor strolled in, his beeper blaring, and your newfound love split for the greener pastures of medical companionship?

Or maybe the last time you took the bus downtown and noticed all those M.D. plates double-parked outside Saks Fifth Avenue?

Life experiences like these are enough to make all of us think: I, TOO, COULD BE A DOCTOR! But could you really? What would medical school be like? Isn't it hard? How would you get in? How would you *stay* in? Is it really worth the effort? It all boils down to one basic question: Are you really M.D. material?

Are You M.D. Material?

Do you respect life?
Even old people's lives?
Even when you're exhausted?

Does your mother brag about you?
A lot?
To everyone?

Do you want to do something rewarding with your life?
Like save mankind?
And own a Beta Max?

Are you in love?
With a terrific person?
Who would love you even if you weren't a doctor?

Would you ever kill yourself?
If something horrible happened to you?
Like waking up and finding you're a dentist?

Do you think other people are intelligent?
As intelligent as you are?
Really?

1

Do you like to eat?
While dissecting?
Human beings?

Do you work harder than everyone you know?
Do you remind them of this?
Every day?

You can relate to these concepts? Maybe you *are* M.D. material. But do you have a *realistic* idea of what being a doctor really means, day to day? Are your social, political, emotional, economic, and medical attitudes what they should be? If you're still uncertain, the following quiz should help you.

Reality Testing: The Facts of Life and Practice as Perceived by Doctors

---

Complete the sentence.

1. Socialized medicine
   a. will result in the equitable distribution of health care.
   b. will result in a medical system as efficient as the U.S. Postal Service, and twice as deadly.
   c. is a Threat to the American Way of Life.
   d. is both b and c.

2. Starting up a practice in today's economic climate
   a. can be successful if the doctor is competent and works hard.
   b. is as easy as pulling impacted wisdom teeth.
   c. is as easy as getting through Customs in Miami with a kilo.
   d. is both b and c.

3. After completing an office visit, most patients will
   a. thank you for your time and wise advice, start on the low-cholesterol diet you've given them, throw away their cigarettes, and pay the receptionist as they leave.
   b. casually inform the secretary that their insurance has lapsed and they won't be able to pay the bill. Ever.
   c. remind you that they know a lawyer uptown. Not that you've done anything wrong. Yet.
   d. both b and c.

4. Analogies

Surgeon is to major metropolitan area as
  a. fish is to water.
  b. sardine is to can.
  c. commuter is to Long Island Expressway.
  d. Dolly Parton is to 32AA bra.

Insurance forms are to practice as
  a. billing is to business.
  b. gridlock is to traffic.
  c. monkey wrench is to machinery.
  d. knees are to Joe Namath.

Malpractice lawyers are to doctors as
  a. fireman is to policeman.
  b. Vichy, France is to the Resistance.
  c. James ("Raider of the Last Park") Watt is to the environment.
  d. *Entamoeba histolytica* (intestinal parasite) is to humans.

Key:

If you answered a to everything: You do not think like a doctor. You are either hopelessly naïve or have overdosed on *Marcus Welby* reruns. Pass Go, collect $200, and go directly into social work.

If you answered b and c to most questions: You are appropriately cynical and have some idea of what it is you want to get into: a rat race with big, smart rats.

If you answered d to everything: You are without question already a medical student. Put this book down! Get back to work! You should be ashamed of yourself. What are you doing *wasting* time when you could have been reading something serious? Someone could *die* tomorrow because you weren't up-to-date on your reading. Worse, your professional reputation could be ruined on rounds tomorrow morning by a question about renal failure. You never really *did* understand renal failure all that well, did you?

The Medical College Survival Aptitude Test

You still want to be a doctor? Even though you realize that after four years of unbelievably expensive medical school you'll face five to seven years of grueling residency at a salary less than the minimum hourly wage?

And even though the only place that will still need young doctors like you after those ten long years of training will be somewhere outside Lubbock, Texas? *Outside* Lubbock, mind you.

Okay. You say you can handle all of these dubious considerations. But how will you fare on the notorious and terrifying MCSAT, whose very initials strike terror in the hearts of pre-meds nationwide? No, we're not talking about the MCATs (Medical College Aptitude Test); everyone knows that that's a piece of cake. What could be simpler than a couple of hundred questions testing how well you can dredge up memories of high-school science class? We're talking about the Medical College *Survival* Aptitude Test.

And, by the way, those of you who answered *a* on "The Facts of Life" test better not take this one. You'll fail it. In any case, this is a weeder course, and you, my friend, have been weeded. Soft hearts and idealistic goals have no place in American medicine. Go enroll in Sociology 101 instead. Social work needs you!

Instructions for Taking the Medical College Survival Aptitude Test

Warning! If you are seen giving or receiving assistance during this examination, the proctor will shoot your hands off!

Warning! Do not eat, drink, smoke, move, or breathe during this examination!

Warning! You may not leave the room for any reason during the examination! If you must leave for bodily functions (which must be verified by the proctor), an armed guard will accompany you to the appropriate restroom!

START ONLY WHEN YOU ARE TOLD TO START!
IF YOU SO MUCH AS GLANCE AT THE TEST BOOKLET BEFORE YOU ARE SPECIFICALLY TOLD TO DO SO, YOUR ENTIRE FUTURE IS RUINED AND YOU MIGHT AS WELL ENROLL IN THE ACE SCHOOL OF TRUCK DRIVING!

Are you ready?

1. **Your favorite activity on weekends is**
   a. studying.
   b. going to study group.

   c. stealing notes from other study groups.
   d. Weekend? What's a weekend?

2. To add variety to your life, you
   a. study in the law library instead of the medical library.
   b. study in the hospital cafeteria.
   c. change tables in the library.
   d. get wild and take an unscheduled fifteen-minute study break.

3. When faced with 150 pages of Microbiology, 60 pages of Pharmacology, 3 sets of slides for Pathology, and a history and physical examination write-up, all assigned Friday and due Monday, you would
   a. cry.
   b. cram the Micro, get last year's cribsheet for Pharm, copy your physical diagnosis partner's write-up word for word, and punt the Pathology assignment completely because you've got a reasonable margin of safety from the last exam. Then go out drinking.
   c. stay up for thirty-six straight hours reading every single word of the assignment and taking impeccable notes, and then oversleep Monday morning, missing the pop quiz that could have gotten you honors.
   d. heave a grateful sigh and say, "Thank God! Finally a light weekend. Now I can catch up on last week's work!"

4. You know medical school will be expensive. You plan to finance your education by
   a. savings, loans, working part-time, some support from parents.
   b. depleting all of the above in the first year when you discover that federal loans are as rare as honest lawyers; resorting to selling yourself as a human guinea pig for unpleasant medical experimentation, living in squalor with four roommates, and selling stolen Quaaludes from the hospital pharmacy.
   c. signing your life (or at least most of your thirties) away to the military, and hoping like hell things stay under control in the Middle East.
   d. giving up the struggle, borrowing at 19 percent so you can feed your kids, and resigning yourself to lifelong debt.

5. You are sitting in the nurses' station at General Hospital. A patient staggers by, vomiting. Your immediate reaction is:

a. you have trouble keeping down your own lunch, but quickly run to the patient to ascertain that nothing is seriously wrong.

b. you tell a nurse to clean up the mess, talk to the patient, and tell you if anything is wrong.

c. you don't notice anything unusual and keep working on the charts.

d. you say to the doctor sitting next to you, "Hey, good thing I didn't wash these pants last night! That's the second time today I've gotten splashed. Gee, that reminds me, I haven't eaten yet today. Anyone up for lunch?"

6. The last time you had a date was

a. graduation night, from college, three years ago.

b. graduation night, from high school, seven years ago.

c. You've never actually had a date, but you certainly plan to have one, as soon as you get some free time.

d. Date? What's a date?

Key:

If you answered a, b, c: You are without a doubt a killer pre-med and have all the lovable characteristics of a great white shark, which will serve you well in medical school.

If you answered d to anything: You medical students! Still reading this! *Surely* you have more important things to do! Have you done that reading on renal failure yet?

If you are looking at this key before doing the test: You pre-meds just don't stop, do you?

If you kept looking for "None of the above" for an answer: Whew! Did I ever save you a lot of time and effort! You have an originality and a need for flexibility that would drive you crazy in the lockstep world of medical education.

If you feel intimidated by the enormity of this venture: Keep reading. It gets worse!

Secrets of the Medical Fraternity
How to Get Immediate Attention in the
Emergency Room

Whether you're in for a tetanus shot, a cut finger, or a stomachache that has bothered you for days, there is one absolutely sure-fire way to get prompt medical attention (and to circumvent the Valkyries who want everything from your last IRS short form to your insurance agent's home phone number):

1. Gasp for breath
2. Clutch your chest
3. Turn blue
4. Stop breathing

A doctor will appear immediately. Of course, he'll be ticked off when you sheepishly hold up your little finger cut, but you *will* see him promptly.

Caution! Perform maneuvers 1 through 4 *only* in private suburban hospitals. If you try this at a big metropolitan hospital, one of the following will happen:

1. Great—you stop breathing, but no one *notices*. You get trampled by the harried ambulance crews that come through every five minutes.

2. As you lie supine on the Emergency Room floor, you are relieved of your watch and wallet by a fellow patient; when you resist, he whips out a Saturday Night special and suddenly your priority changes from LOW to STAT. You get seen, not for the cut on your finger, but for the gunshot wound in your chest.

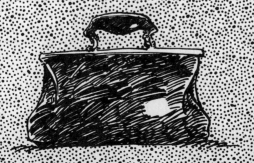

CHAPTER 2

How to Get into Medical School, or, Don't Believe Them When They Say "There Is No Right Answer to This Question"

What Are the Medical Schools Looking for, Anyway?

Jimmy Stewart.

John Glenn.

Henry Fonda.

Medical-school admissions committees basically comprise white, middle-aged, conservative, male members of the ruling elite. They do not like loud feminists, members of the counterculture, or anyone who doesn't regularly vote Republican. The interview is not the place to mention your support of Jane Fonda's trip to Hanoi, the teachings of some obscure guru from Nepal, or the Ayatollah.

The admissions committees are looking for five basic characteristics: *intelligence, tenacity, ability to work with others, self-motivation, compassion* (see chart). Those excessively discussed items—grade point average, MCAT scores, and published papers—are simply quantifiable measurements of the Ideal Potential Doctor. Schools pay an inordinate amount of attention to these markers because they make comparison of candidates easier. Of course, the numbers don't represent any *real* difference—who knows whether a 3.4 GPA from Stanford in Physics is a better potential doctor than a 3.8 from the University of Michigan in English?—but it at least

1. Intelligence: The ability to read, assimilate, and regurgitate vast quantities of medical information. No one wants a doctor who says, "Uh, gee—I'll tell you what you've got as soon as I can go look it up, okay?"

2. Tenacity: The ability to *keep* reading, assimilating, and regurgitating vast quantities of medical information without demanding reason for doing so, plus the ability to work thirty-six hours straight without questioning the rationale of this training.

3. Ability to Work with Others: This actually translates into the ability to manipulate others into cheerfully doing what you want them to do, regardless of their own best interests. This ability is first utilized in convincing the admissions committee to accept you; later, you will hone this skill on nurses, orderlies, residents, and staff, until you work your way up to chairman of the hospital. Of course, when you're chairman, you don't have to bother convincing them that they *want* to do anything—you just *make* them do it.

4. Self-motivation: How guilty are you about free time? Do you feel that time not spent in a goal-oriented activity is wasted time? Do you wish your parents had sent you to science camp, not tennis camp? After you spend Sunday afternoon sailing, do you wish you had stayed home and read instead? Do you check at school the next day to make sure everyone else took off Sunday afternoon? When they all say that they did, do you worry that they are lying? Are you plagued by the fear that people at some other university are working harder than you and getting ahead? You are obviously prime medical school material—or a candidate for the Funny Farm!

5. Compassion: Compassion is a terrific thing to pay lip service to (after all, who wants to claim that they *don't* train compassionate doctors?), but impossible to measure. Therefore, aside from a few ridiculous essays you might be asked to write, giving "Examples of what a compassionate and moral person I am," no one will ask or be interested in this aspect of your personality. And frankly, it's probably the least important of the five critical characteristics. Would you rather have a doctor who holds your hands compassionately as you expire from pneumonia, or an unpleasant jerk who treats and cures you with the latest antibiotic?

gives the admissions committees some hard numbers to point to.

What If You Just Don't Have the Grades; or, How to Interview

What can you do if you have MCATs in the negative numbers and a series of debacles in Organic Chemistry splattered across your transcript? What can you do if your transcript is to your application as a gunshot wound is to the chest (unquestionably damaging, quite possibly fatal, but—with good management—sometimes salvageable)? You must seize the moment, of course, and sparkle at the interview!

The medical-school admissions committee regards the interview as a routine procedure that reassures them you are alert, well-oriented, and capable of meaningful speech. The interview gives them a chance to ascertain that you are able to *act* normal for periods of up to fifteen minutes, that you had some role in writing your application (or at least you are familiar with its content), and that you, like every other applicant, look uncomfortable in a suit and have unpleasantly clammy hands.

But! Those of you with force of personality coupled with a weak academic track record must seize this opportunity to impress upon the committee what an *interesting* addition you'd make to the class, how *unique* you are, and how you would add *depth* and *variety* to the freshman class they are now assembling.

Here, then, are a few suggested interviewing gambits for the truly desperate:

The New Nixon. It worked for him, why not for you? Bring up that embarrassing topic, your awful grades, but point out that *then* (all two semesters ago) you were young and foolish, but now you are older, serious, and dedicated (at least definitely older). Show them how your grades this semester in Comparative Film are *much* better than those unfortunate Chemistry grades of last year.

My school is tough, really tough. Explain that your school is a very academically rigid school, not a grade factory like Harvard, where grade inflation results in half the class with A's and the other with A−'s. Pine Manor really made you *work* for those D's.

My grades are bad but my heart is pure; or, my mission in Bear's Paw, West Virginia. Look extremely sincere (try imitating a bassett hound) and explain that all you want is to dedicate your life to a poor, underprivileged area without TV reception, running water, or even a Bloomie's. Talk about how thrilled you would be to work as the town's only family practitioner, providing obstetric, medical, and psychiatric care day and night, 365 days a year, for remuneration of hog bellies, tobacco sheaves, and hearty thanks. Keep looking sincere. It also helps if you have ever ventured afield from your native metropolitan area to visit some rural location (and, no, wintering in Gstaad doesn't count); it will sound fairly unconvincing if you tell the admissions committee that you know you'll love country life because you've never missed an episode of *The Waltons*.

I'll do anything! This may work if you are young, pretty, and actually will do anything. A similar approach, "Sir, I couldn't help but notice that you are in serious need of a new motor vehicle. Perhaps a Porsche," may also work. But again, only if you can deliver.

I'm at the end of my rope . . . and I've got a gun! Very risky. Probably only of short-term benefit. ("Here, put on this white coat—of course we want you in our medical school—the sleeves buckle in front. Of course you're a medical student, just go along with these nice men.") Used by those who think that shooting an admissions officer is a great way to impress Jodie Foster.

Interviewing the Interviewers: Loaded Questions Aimed at You

Interviewers are tricky people. Year after year they see cattle cars of anxiety-racked pre-meds crossing their doorsteps; they're a lot more experienced than you and they have a lot less to lose. Some favor the all-out assault, the ever-popular stress interview that starts with a handshake and then immediately launches into "What a lousy academic record! What makes you think you're capable of making life-determining decisions? You can't even get an A in Physiology! Why did you apply to medical school?"

Others favor the "I'm your friend" interview, during which they probe your deepest darkest secrets: "So tell me more about this problem with your girlfriend—she decided not to come down for your interview, eh? Will her career always take precedence? You think she'll be able to give you emotional support?"

But most of the interviews are usually of the low-key, "Tell us a little about yourself, about why you want to be a doctor" type. Watch out, however, for the following time-bomb questions, which might be better answered without, shall we say, *complete* candor:

1. What are your weaknesses?

Now, *really!* It's *their* job to ferret out your weaknesses. Why should you make it easy for them? Say something, but remember the McCarthy era and tell them something they already know. Don't dredge up further character flaws. Mention perhaps that crummy string of Invertebrate Neuroanatomy grades sitting right in front of him on your transcript. Remember, they're looking for reasons to flip you into the REJECT pile—why give them ammunition?

And if you really must say something, make it sickeningly sweet and extroverted, like "My greatest flaw is to give so much of myself to others that my own life is sometimes compromised. This, I am sure, will make me a better doctor, though."

2. What is your most essential possession?

Do not be flip.

Answering "My Bloomingdale's charge card" will get you labeled materialistic.

Answering "My husband" will get you pegged as a tad possessive.

You might be thought serious, if a little narrow-minded, if you mentioned your microscope or Lehninger's *Biochemistry* text.

A perennial standby—the Bible —can never hurt.

Do not under any circumstances mention your inflatable sex toys.

3. What cause would you die for?

Don't say, "Getting into medical school." It's one thing to *be* desperate, and quite another to *sound* it.

4. Explain exactly why your grades fell so abruptly one term.

The interviewer doesn't really want to know the messy details of your sordid social life, and how they impacted on your academic work, so don't tell him. Do *not* get into the intimate details of how Elaine dumped you, and then you got herpes from her best friend, and then she wanted a reconciliation . . . no, no, no.

Say: "I was in a deep coma that entire term."

Don't say: "I was in a clinical depression and couldn't cope."

Say: "I was working sixty hours a week as a short-order cook to provide for my aging parents, and donating my free time to the Red Cross."

Don't say: "Well, that was the term that my cocaine use just got out of control, I guess."

Give a short, succinct answer that would not embarrass you if you told it to your aunt Margie. And emphasize that the terrible grades were strictly environment-related and will *not* happen again.

5. Who else has interviewed you?

Uh, oh! They *know* you're a borderline candidate. They want to know who else has gambled on you. If the only other school that has answered your letters is the Oshkosh School of Medicine and Barbering Sciences, you have one of two options. 1) Keep quiet, or 2) lie. Say "Harvard" confidently. You think they're going to check? They aren't. But they will put your application in the "brilliant and creative, but erratic grades" file, instead of in the "bad grades" file. After all, if Harvard interviewed you, you *must* be okay.

6. How do you plan to raise a family?

Suffice it to say that men are never asked this question. If you are a woman, you will be labeled a radical feminist if you reply in an enraged tone, "You're *not* allowed to ask me that question." Telling them that you had a hysterectomy so children wouldn't interfere with your love affair with medicine will get you labeled intense, but strange. Asking the interviewer how *he* plans to raise *his* family is daring but risky. You'll be labeled a card-carrying troublemaker—and uppity, to boot.

Just take a deep breath, suppress an impulse to phone the ACLU, and give the standard answer. "I know medical school will be time-consuming, and that raising a family will take a lot of organization and effort, but I'm *not* going to leave medicine when the first baby comes."

Six Indications That the Interview Is Going Down the Drain: Warning Signs That You're Going to Have to Study Anatomy in Spanish, or Not at All

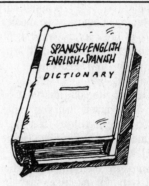

1. Before the interview, you see the secretary carrying your folder into the committee. Loud, uncontrolled laughter emits from the room.

2. As the interview starts, the folder is passed among the three physicians interviewing you. You notice that COURTESY INTERVIEW: OUR UNDERGRADUATE SCHOOL is stamped in large red letters on the folder.

3. The first interviewer flips through briefly, tosses your application on the table, leans forward, and says, "Let's not waste everyone's time."

4. The second interviewer asks in a friendly fashion what your alternative career plans are. When you reply that you haven't made any, he strongly suggests that you do.

5. The third interviewer looks at your MCAT scores and audibly gasps. "Christ—I haven't seen scores like this in years! What did you do, fall asleep?"

6. As you walk out the door, the interviewer says, "Well, I hope you didn't waste, uh, *spend* too much money getting down here..."

What to Do If You Don't (God Forbid!) Get into Medical School

1. Cry.

2. Telephone relatives in the Mafia capable of applying selected pressure.

3. Surrender $800 to Stanley Kaplan and take the MCATs again. And again. And again.

4. Reevaluate the medical schools you applied to. Did you apply only to the ten most competitive medical schools in the country, mistakenly believing that you wouldn't settle for the U. of Ohio at Athens no matter what?

5. Reevaluate your interview behavior. Did you tell them you wanted to practice dermatology in a medically underserved area like Georgetown? Did you insult them by saying that you were interviewing at their school only for practice, and that you really weren't interested in spending your valuable time training at a rinky-dink operation like the University of Cincinnati? *Helpful hint for the future:* Don't do these things.

6. Reevaluate your career plans. Maybe getting a PhD in Biology and studying slimy invertebrates the rest of your life won't be so bad. Or you could go into malpractice law and make everyone who *did* get in damned sorry that they did, and you didn't.

7. Brush up on your Spanish. Or Italian. Or Filipino. Jarvik, inventor of the artificial heart, did it, and so can you. As long as your parents have the cash for tuition and annual "contributions" required by many foreign medical schools, and you don't mind spending four or five years in the Mexican back country cramming Physiology and Biochemistry in a foreign language, then coming back to practice in the U.S., where comments will be made daily behind your back. This is *not* exactly the path of least resistance, and is really recommended only to those with great mental — and intestinal — fortitude.

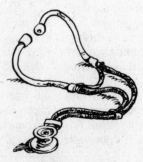

CHAPTER 3

Acting Like a Doctor

From the first day of your acceptance to medical school to your last dying breath, you are officially (at least in the eyes of others) A DOCTOR! Never mind that you don't know a thing about saving lives yet. Your relationships with everyone—from your mom and dad to that good-looker in the singles bar—will change.

It's as if with medical-studenthood automatically comes medical expertise. Suddenly everyone regards you as a medical authority and a source of free advice about any subject even distantly related to medicine. People will solemnly ask you—whether you are a junior medical student, a staff obstetrician, or a world-famous researcher—should they have their hernia repaired now? Should Aunt Mamie be sent to a nursing home? How do you open those child-resistant bottles without damaging your teeth? And what's this about Tylenol killing people, anyway—isn't that the pain-reliever more hospitals use?

Getting the respect due an authority is fun. But actually fielding the questions is a pain. As a "doctor," you must be particularly wary of falling into the Cocktail-party Consult trap and of exposing yourself to the Attack on the Entire American Medical Establishment, Including You, Its Most Readily Available Representative. If you think well on your feet, the following advice should help you deflect these assaults and still be invited back to cocktail parties.

The Cocktail-party Consult

You may be sitting on the beach. You may be at the family Thanksgiving table. You may be engrossed in a fascinating discussion of Turkish land reform with a Tom Selleck look-alike. Wherever you are, you can be sure you're *not* in a hospital or a doctor's office. Suddenly, someone sashays up to you, and with utmost confidence and absolutely no reticence launches into a loud and graphic discussion of the recent disruption of his or her intimate bodily function: hemorrhoids, interrupted pregnancy, peptic ulcer, bloody stool. As a doctor, you are expected to:

1. be enthralled (after all, this *is* your business).

2. comment intelligently on the problem (for free, of course).
3. critique the care their physician has provided.

You would like nothing better than to rejoin the group that is now animatedly discussing the Balkan wars (and grab the Tom Selleck look-alike, who is putting on his coat and heading out the door). But the complainer is now directly facing you, waiting for a response to his tirade about the failing and aging mechanisms of his not particularly interesting body.

You have three options:

1. Feel stupid but plead the truth. "Mr. Rothspot, I'm an ophthalmologist, not a urologist. I'm sure that if your urologist feels you need your prostate operated on, he must be right." Of course, Mr. Rothspot will not respond well to your answer; he will think that he has wasted his time on a willful ignoramus, or else he will think that you are deliberately withholding your opinion because you are stingy and want to be paid. Either way, he'll feel slighted, you'll feel dumb, and the Tom Selleck look-alike will leave—and not with you.

2. Be earnest and play it safe. Put on your professional listening look (you'll have this look perfected by the time you finish medical school), ask a few perfunctory questions, and then give a careful non-opinion, something along the lines of "Well, Mrs. Graves, if those big bulging eyes are really bothering you, then I think you should schedule an appointment with your family doctor as soon as possible." Mrs. Graves will be pleased because you've taken an interest in her fascinating (to her) problem and have given her a medical opinion (of sorts). And you're safe because you've told her to see a doctor; so you're covered if there really *is* something wrong with her. (You will find yourself taking this safe but boring route as you accumulate more tangible assets.)

3. Be wildly irresponsible. Fight back! Start a crusade against the cheapskates of the world who won't see a doctor the proper way and who are ruining your social life. Don't let them prey on your guilt to get help!

Diagnose terrible diseases from their vague descriptions. "You've been feeling really cold? And slowing down a lot recently? You've got terminal moraine. You need a doctor immediately!"

Or wait until the cheapskate in question has finished his litany of woes. Look completely blank. Then say, "Oh, *now* I get it! You have me confused with my sister the *gastroenterologist. I'm* a poli-sci major at Barnard. And you've reminded me *exactly* why I didn't go into medicine. Yuck!"

Or try this: "Mr. Crohn, can I be frank with you? That's the most disgusting set of symptoms I've ever heard. Please excuse me."

Or laugh uncontrollably and call all your friends over by yelling, "Hey guys! This is a story you've got to hear. This guy hasn't gotten it up for years." (That'll be the last time he asks for free advice.)

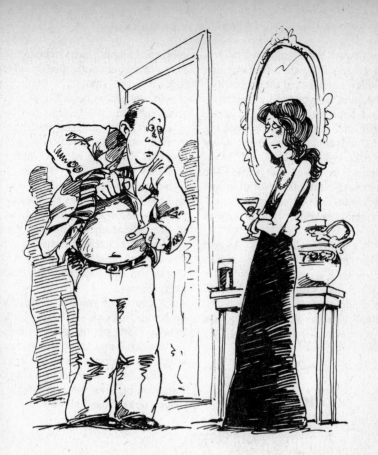

Or pull the person into the kitchen and tell them you must perform a biopsy before you could give any kind of opinion. But since your services are free, you'll have to use a kitchen knife and skimp on the local anesthesia.

But if you want to protect yourself from people seeking free opinions, but want to continue to practice medicine in the United States, you can always look at the cheapskate coldly, hand them your business card, and tell them that they can call during office hours. Don't expect to get invited back to dinner, though.

Warding Off Attacks on the Entire American Medical Establishment—and You, Its most Readily Available Representative

A good time to laugh and say, "Oh, I'm not a *people* surgeon, I'm a *tree* surgeon."

Otherwise, very difficult to deflect.

People with a grudge against

doctors will launch into an attack on all doctors once they find out that you are a member of the profession. They will tell you wildly inaccurate third-hand stories about vicious, cruel, incompetent doctors with big fees and cold stethoscopes; every mistake and every delay will be attributed to *intent,* not error. The American public has a lot of hostility toward doctors, and you will undoubtedly bear the brunt of some of it.

It's a no-win situation. As part of the medical fraternity, you naturally have a general sympathy for doctors, and your first reaction will be in defense of your colleagues. "Really," you will say in your most calm and rational voice, "there must be more to this story; perhaps the facts are not straight." This, of course, will only enrage the person attacking you, who wants you to agree completely with him that these terrible doctors are greedy and careless and should be sued for every cent they have.

Nor should you fall back on such antagonizing statements as "Clearly you have absolutely no idea of what you are talking about, and until you do, I have no interest in discussing this or any other case with you," unless you are fond of loud, and angry battles.

Of course, if you are interested in being welcome at next year's family Thanksgiving get-together, the most rational response to any attack on American medicine is to say, "Hmmmm. That's quite a story. I *must* go back for more of this delicious turkey," and slip away.

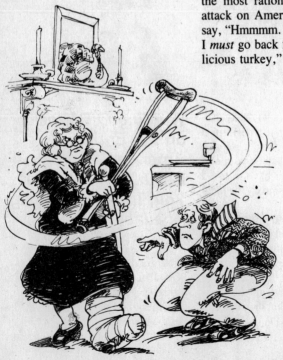

CHAPTER 4

So What's Medical School Really Like? or, In the Fundus of the Beast

Quiz:

1. What's the difference between a medical student and a pile of dog poop?
   a. No one intentionally steps on dog poop.
   b. No one goes *out of their way* to step on dog poop.
   c. What's the similarity?

2. Four years of medical school is like
   a. eight years in Folsom Prison.
   b. eight years in Folsom Prison for a crime you didn't commit.
   c. graduate school in any of the sciences.

Key:
If you answered a or b: You are a medical student. You are still reading this. And you *still* haven't read up on renal failure. Don't think it won't catch up with you!
If you answered c: Keep reading. *You're* in for a surprise.

Rosie Ruiz Medical School Survival Tactics

---

1. Don't waste time in class. Beg, borrow, or steal notes.

2. Don't waste time trying to figure out what's important. Look at last year's exams. Ask the prof what his research is on. No matter how obscure, it will be on the final examination.

3. Don't waste time in lab. Why kill time waiting for chemicals to react in a predictable way? Just figure out how they're supposed to react, and why.

How to Succeed in Medical School Without Really Trying

You can't.

The first day of medical school is the most anxiety-producing. You look around and wonder if you are surrounded by geniuses. Don't worry. You aren't. You wonder if you have been admitted by mistake, and if, after you fall flat on your face in the first examination, you will be used as Exhibit One for why the admissions policy should be changed. Don't worry. You won't

flunk out. You can't. Medical school is a lot like Alcatraz—no one leaves until his time is up.

But remember: *Medical school is a marathon, not a sprint;* take a tip from Rosie Ruiz and ride the subway while your classmates run.

Your Classmates, and Other Congenital Anomalies

Your classmates will be an interesting and eclectic bunch, quite different from the cookie-cutter white, middle-class male Republicans of yesteryear. Political attitudes range from those who view Planned Parenthood as a Communist threat, to Social Democrats lobbying for Socialized Medicine, to the simply selfish who favor Reaganomics because it ensures future possession of a two-car garage and the BMWs to fill it. Heated political discussions in the halls are not unusual, and are punctuated by cutting statements such as "They're not going to give *you* an M.D.—you're going to get a 007 license!"

The Doctor's Kid Who Would Rather Be a Poet. He's been pressured since fifth grade to be a doctor. "I don't want to force you into a career decision," Dr. Daddy says. "You can be any kind of doctor you want." The Doctor's Kid is never really sure *why* he's in medical school; after listening to Dad's epic tales of his own medical-school ex-

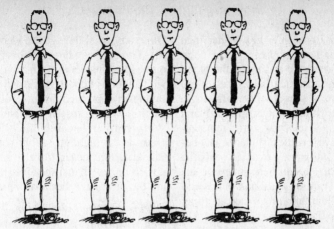

THE MEDICAL SCHOOL CLASS OF YESTERYEAR

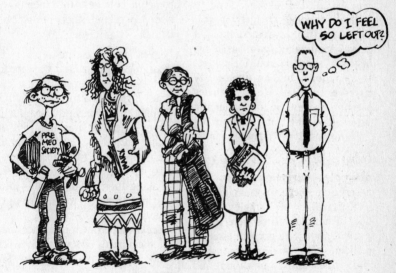

WHY DO I FEEL SO LEFT OUT?

PRE MED SOCIETY

THE MEDICAL SCHOOL CLASS OF TODAY

periences, actually *being* there is, well, anticlimactic and a little dull. Most likely to step out for a few years, be a Peace Corps worker in the Dominican Republic, and dis-cover that *that* isn't so interesting, either. He'll come back to medical school eventually, and go into Anesthesia or Hospital Administration.

The Paramedic Vet. Older than most of the class, he served in 'Nam as a paramedic and loved the blood 'n' guts so much he decided to go to medical school. He wears jungle gear to class, looks grizzled and tough, and tells war stories that nauseate even medical students. But beneath that grizzly exterior beats the heart of a teddy bear—despite his macho talk of gunshot wounds and multiple trauma, he winds up going into Pediatrics.

The Overeducated Dilettante. He already has a J.D. and an M.A. in English Lit. He says he came to medical school to perfect his golf game—at first, everyone thought he was kidding. Rumor has it his trust fund supports him. He's a terrible student, but he eventually passes everything. His classmates love him because he throws terrific parties. Residents don't like him because he just doesn't give a damn.

The Former Flower Child. A bit older than her classmates—she marched in the anti-Vietnam war demonstrations in Berkeley when most of her classmates were in the seventh grade. She got interested in medicine after working in a free clinic. She believes in natural and holistic alternatives to medicine, and struggles to enlighten her classmates. Most of them, however, are as interested in looking at their own cervixes as they are in looking at their own tonsils—not very.

The Self-appointed Upholder of the Protestant Work Ethic. A nice but very dull and humorless woman. On a rare social outing, she went to see *Tootsie* and laughed exactly once. Most frequently seen standing with a group of chortling classmates saying in a puzzled way, "I don't get it." She makes an outstanding study partner because the study group is the highlight of her social calendar. She never forgets, she's always prepared, and she loves having the meeting at her apartment.

Paranoid Pete, Victim of the Premed Syndrome. Pete, extremely bright but hopelessly paranoid, was warped forever by the Pre-med Syndrome in college. He's incredibly good at psyching others out and he just can't stop himself. He:

- leaves textbooks around the library open to material way ahead of the class assignment, with a few lines highlighted for authenticity, hoping to impress professors and drive other students into fits of panic when they see how far ahead he is (he doesn't realize that they saw his covert distribution and are shaking their heads sadly—they are not strangers to the Pre-med Syndrome).
- checks all pertinent references out of the library and uses them for doorstops in his apartment for months.
- purposely puts mistakes into the lecture notes he transcribes for the class note service, and tells only his friends about the planted errors (of course, classmates who attended the lecture catch the errors and threaten him with permanent bodily harm should he ever do this again).

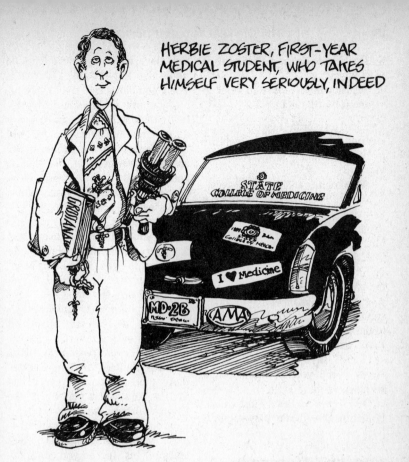

HERBIE ZOSTER, FIRST-YEAR MEDICAL STUDENT, WHO TAKES HIMSELF VERY SERIOUSLY, INDEED

Fortunately you won't have to put up with Paranoid Pete for four years. He'll have a nervous breakdown after short-circuiting his body's stress system, and drop out. The last you'll hear of him, he'll be recuperating in a Tucson health spa, planning to write an exposé of American Medicine.

The Class Clown. Day one, freshman year, he arrives late to class, looks around, and says in slack-jawed amazement, "Hey! Waaaait a second! This doesn't sound like law school."

The White Knight of Medicine. A few humorless folk will be "Answering a Calling," not just training for a job like the rest of us. These people are easy to spot; day one of first year they will do at least three of the following:
1. Join the AMA
2. Put a medical-school sticker on the car.
3. Get vanity license plates that say "MD2B."
4. Buy caduceus tiepins, key chains, and belt buckles.
5. Subscribe to the *New England Journal of Medicine.*

6. Pontificate on the difficult life of a physician.
7. Instruct their spouse to refer to them as "the doctor."

The acid test for those who are "Answering a Calling" is the inability to find the humor in the following vignette:

A doctor dies and goes to Heaven.

At St. Peter's Gate he finds a long line. As is his custom, he rushes to the front. However, St. Peter turns him back and asks him to wait in line, just like everyone else.

Slightly disgruntled, he rejoins the end of the line. Moments later, a white-haired man with white coat, stethoscope, and black bag rushes to the front of the line, waves to St. Peter, and is immediately admitted.

"Hey!" says the doctor angrily. "How come you let *him* through without waiting?"

"Oh," says St. Peter, "that's God. Sometimes he likes to play doctor."

Fun and Games in Gross Anatomy Lab; or, Gross Is the Time, the Place, the Emotion, Gross Is the Way We Are Feeling

Gross Anatomy will dominate your life during freshman year of medical school, for better or worse. Usually for worse. The cadaver smells worse and worse as the year progresses. Though you will become accustomed to the smell after a time, that clinging, pervasive odor will have only negative effects on your love life. Eau de Cadavre is not a popular scent!

Anatomy is overwhelming, albeit essential for a doctor to know all the muscles, bones, nerves, and blood vessels in the human body, and how they connect, disconnect, and originally form. At first, mastering Anatomy seems just about as manageable as someone handing you the New York City subway map and telling you to memorize every stop and every connection by Friday. By *Friday,* mind you, because on Monday you're starting on the Los Angeles Freeway system!

A few pointers for making Anatomy more fun than memorizing all of the R's in Webster's Seventh:

1. Pick good-looking dissection partners. At least you'll have *something* nice to look at every day in lab. And when you get to the Living/Surface Anatomy section, your cheap thrills are guaranteed— that's when your tennis-star partner takes off his shirt so you can study the rippling muscles of his chest wall and back, and squeeze his pectoralis major and minor, serratus anterior, latissimus dorsi . . . for *educational* purposes, of course!

2. If you can't get good-looking, settle for partners who are married. Married students who will take pity on you and invite you over for a home-cooked meal are worth their weight in gold, especially to the struggling first-year student whose stomach still rebels at the sight, sound, or smell of hospital cafeteria food.

3. Never study in the lab late at

night by yourself. Creepy is not the word for six dead people and you alone in a room. Such an experience does *not* enhance cardiac stability, especially if you have practical-joker dissection partners who favor stunts such as startling you with a tap from a cadaver hand, or hiding under a dissection table and whispering in a thin, quavering voice, "Help . . . me . . . I'm still . . . alive . . ."

4. Remember that dissection requires some degree of skill and forethought. A now-infamous group of medical students of a major eastern medical center had neither. These individuals, future psychiatrists all, cheerfully hacked their way through delicate structures until even the venerable department chairman, who literally wrote the book, was unable to identify anything. "Well, kids,"

he'd say, shaking his head, "I suppose this was the brachial plexus. Doesn't look like much, all shredded up, does it? What are you using, scalpels or buzz saws? They did cleaner work in *The Texas Chainsaw Massacre.*"

In the first year of medical school, you learn how things work: Physiology, Anatomy, Biochemistry. In the second year, you learn how things go wrong: Pathology, Introduction to Human Illness, Psychiatry, Microbiology, Pharmacology. To help you get away from it all, the end of second year is punctuated by a marathon examination that lasts two days and covers two years of work: the National Boards—Part I. Only then do you get to make the break from the classroom and move to where the action is, the hospital.

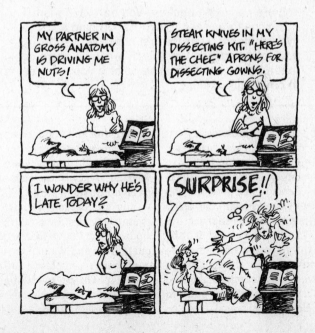

Exam: National Boards—Part 1

QUESTION 1: A man wants toast for breakfast.
a. He has a .3 percent chance of fatal electric shock if the toaster he uses was built before the 1972 Uniform Toaster Standards (Epidemiology).
b. His risk of botulism is significantly greater should he choose canned strawberry jam instead of bottled elderberry, because bottled elderberry is more acidic (Microbiology).
c. His risk of divorce in the next decade is significantly greater should his wife not habitually join him for breakfast, according to the 1920 landmark study by Dr. J. Kay (Psychiatry).
d. The median age of death for unmarried males in Afghanistan is thirty-eight (Left Field).

Answer in the following format:
1. a and c are true.
2. b and d are true.
3. a, b, and c are true.
4. d is true.
5. all are true.
6. you are panicking because you have 350 more questions to answer in this session, and it just took you five minutes to *read* the first question.
7. you are wondering just exactly what you were doing for the last two years, because nothing you know seems to be on this exam.

The National Boards cast a giant shadow over the second year. Two days of solid questions, forty-five seconds for each question, supervised by Gestapo-like proctors who hover like vultures over your seats, certain that given the slightest opportunity, you—you, who will be entrusted with people's *lives* the next day—would cheat. They confiscate your coat and purse (you might have *Lehninger's Biochemistry* copied in minuscule writing sewed into the lining), and seat you far away from your untrustworthy cohorts.

But it's all worth it, you think to yourself, because as soon as the Boards are over—presto, change-o! —you are suddenly transformed overnight into a third-year medical student. And you'll go into the hospital! Onto the wards! In a white coat! With a stethoscope and everything! It will be so exciting! It's amazing how convincing the enthusiasm of youth can be.

CHAPTER 5

Strangers in a Strange Land: Medical Students on the Hospital Wards

Never get sick in July!

July 1st in a hospital is like December 7th in Pearl Harbor. July 1st is when the new Interns start, when the new Medical Students start, and when Junior Residents are suddenly in charge.

July 1st is when a nurse yells, "Hey, Dr. Parobeck!" but Dr. Parobeck doesn't stop because she's been a doctor for only three days, and no one has ever called her "doctor" before.

July 1st is when the cardiac-arrest bell goes off and three floors initiate the fire-drill evacuation.

July 1st is when the senior staff plan to stay up all night.

July 1st is utter chaos.

Into this maelstrom wanders our hero, the freshly minted, wide-eyed third-year student, decked out in his spanking new white coat with six (working) pens, a penlight, a note pad, two textbooks, enough medical equipment for a small Yucatán clinic—stethoscope, otolaryngo-scope, reflex hammer, tuning forks, safety pins, pocket vision screeners, sphygmomanometer— (none of which he knows how to use) and with high hopes, extreme anxiety, and an uncertain smile.

In less than a month only the uncertain smile will remain.

The coat will be splattered with God knows what, the pens will have been filched by Residents, the note pad will be scrawled with illegible but no doubt critical data, the textbooks will be stashed in the on-call room (with the first pages of each chapter neatly underlined, marking precisely the point at which the student fell asleep), and the medical equipment will be left at home, where it at least won't be stolen or broken.

And the extreme anxiety? Replaced by the sad discovery that the third-year student is on that part of the totem pole that is embedded in the ground.

How Medical Students Dress for Success

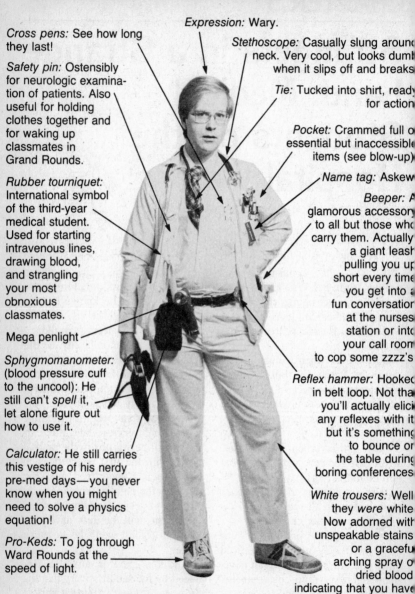

Expression: Wary.

Cross pens: See how long they last!

Safety pin: Ostensibly for neurologic examination of patients. Also useful for holding clothes together and for waking up classmates in Grand Rounds.

Rubber tourniquet: International symbol of the third-year medical student. Used for starting intravenous lines, drawing blood, and strangling your most obnoxious classmates.

Mega penlight

Sphygmomanometer: (blood pressure cuff to the uncool): He still can't *spell* it, let alone figure out how to use it.

Calculator: He still carries this vestige of his nerdy pre-med days—you never know when you might need to solve a physics equation!

Pro-Keds: To jog through Ward Rounds at the speed of light.

Stethoscope: Casually slung around neck. Very cool, but looks dumb when it slips off and breaks.

Tie: Tucked into shirt, ready for action.

Pocket: Crammed full of essential but inaccessible items (see blow-up).

Name tag: Askew

Beeper: A glamorous accessory to all but those who carry them. Actually a giant leash pulling you up short every time you get into a fun conversation at the nurses' station or into your call room to cop some zzzz's.

Reflex hammer: Hooked in belt loop. Not that you'll actually elicit any reflexes with it, but it's something to bounce on the table during boring conferences.

White trousers: Well they *were* white. Now adorned with unspeakable stains or a graceful arching spray of dried blood indicating that you have at least hit, if not stayed in an artery in the recent past.

Note: Pediatricians add decoys to this outfit: Koala bear on stethoscope, squeaky toys in pocket.

Pocket Dissection

A. Breast pocket: High-visibility items which underscore your competence. High accessibility.

Pocket vision screener: Looks nifty and you might even use it.

Pharmaceutical company note pads: Generally covered with illegible scrawls concerning everything from your kid's dental appointment to Mr. Smith's oxygen levels the night he arrested.

Penlight: Always good for brownie points to be the one student with a functioning penlight.

Pens: Carry at least five. Your Residents will filch them from you shamelessly.

Name tag: Nine out of ten doctors surveyed wear them crooked. Gives sense of identity to those with weak ego functions: Encourages Resident not to yell, "Hey, you!"

Handbook: Containing *only* the essential, distilled, absolutely basic principles of Medicine, Surgery, or whatever service you're on. Because that's all you want at 2 A.M.

File cards: Notes on who your patients are, what's wrong with them, what you did to fix it, and whether it's working. *Would* be useful, but is generally illegible, or out-of-date.

Tools for survival: IV equipment, many test tubes, 4 × 4 gauze pads Band-Aids, adhesive tape, lab slips, etc., to start IV's and draw blood. *Also:* Lunch, a mushed banana.

Change: For vending machines where you'll be eating breakfast, lunch, and dinner for the next five years, and for calling home to tell your spouse you're sorry, you'll be late again.

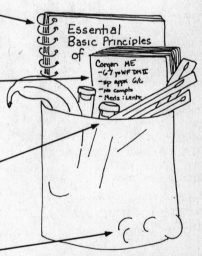

B. Side pocket: Functional tools for daily living. Low accessibility: Impossible to get to most items without disimpacting the entire pocket.

Drawing Blood: Perfecting the Technique

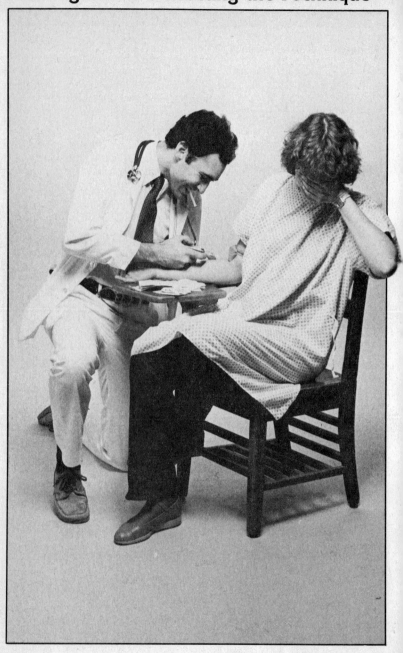

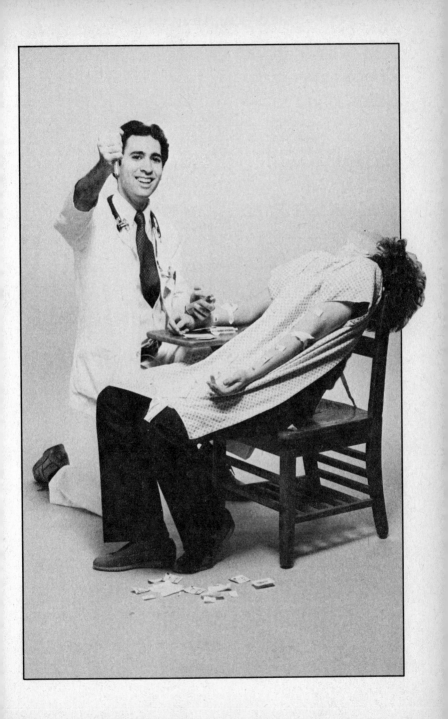

And What's In That Mysterious Black Bag?

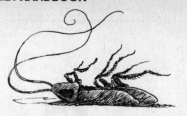

a. Lunch (from yesterday).
b. A change of underwear.
c. A pile of dense untouched reprints from medical journals.

Scut—a Definition

Scut comprises the secretarial and technical aspects of patient care, all the boring tedious jobs that must be done to keep the patients going— starting intravenous lines, drawing blood, filling out insurance forms, locating chest X rays. Scut is whatever the Resident has to do that teaches him nothing. Scut takes up nine-tenths of the hospital day.

Scut—Word Usage

RESIDENT: "Christ! Look at this morning's scut list! Where's that Medical Student?"

STUDENT: "I'd love to go to lecture, but I'm buried alive by scut."

Significant Changes in the Third-Year Medical Student's Life

1. S/He no longer blushes. At anything.

2. S/He can't remember his wife's/girlfriend's (husband's/boyfriend's) name.

3. S/He discovers that it is indeed possible to survive on four hours of sleep a night.

4. The cockroaches in his/her apartment starve to death.

5. S/He masters the art of sleeping on (his/her) feet, eyes wide open.

6. S/He discovers there is no such thing as an interesting case when you haven't slept in thirty-six hours.

The Med-Student Anthem
The Scutpuppy Song*

Oh, I'm a scutpuppy and
  I'm okay!
I work all night and I
  work all day!
I start I.V.'s, I fight
  disease, I take blood
  to the lab-or-tree—
And if I'm really lucky,
  get to bed by 3!

*(To the tune of "I'm a Lumberjack")

Q. What's the difference between an operating-room nurse and a lobster?
A. Most Residents have never eaten lobster.

CHAPTER 6

The Doctor's Social Life, and Other Overrated Phenomena

Being a doctor will drastically change your social life. For men, the medicinal whiff of medical power is the world's greatest aphrodisiac; for women, it is roughly equivalent to the combined scent of skunkweed, old smelts, and musk still on the musk ox.

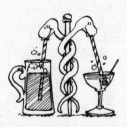

The Social Life of Male Doctors: Face It, You Are a Catch!

You saw it on *Marcus Welby*, or *House Calls*, on *Trapper John, M.D.*, on *M*A*S*H:* Women fall all over doctors. To your surprise and delight, you are suddenly a catch. Girls who dismissed you as a pimply-faced, nerdy pre-med grind will be thrilled to meet you, now that you are a pimply-faced nerdy ear-nose-throat surgeon.

How to Win Friends and Influence Secretaries

Singles' bars, especially the bars nearest the hospital, are the ideal hunting grounds. After all, the secretaries have to know where to find you.

But being in the right place at the right time in such a situation is not enough. Your deportment in the bar is critical. The following four steps will make it completely clear to everyone that you are a doctor:

1. Pay the bartender to say loudly, "Hi, *Doctor* Korsakoff! Here for a few of your usual evening vodkas?"

2. Go with a fellow doctor from the hospital; talk loudly about your cases, dropping terms that the average high-school graduate will recognize as medical. *Good ones to try:* Doctor. Patient. Hospital. Surgery. *Not:* Immunoassay. Agglutination. Electrophoresis. Encephalopathy. Big words like these will only encourage the object of your romantic sights to head straight down the bar to those loud-talking—but English-speaking—lawyers.

3. Wear a beeper conspicuously on your body. Have your buddy page you from the bar telephone by loudly intoning, "Dr. Barfly! Dr. Barfly! Call the Emergency Room!" If the page is garbled, make sure no one thinks you're just a plumber or businessman; say loudly, "Damn! That's the *Emergency Room!*" If it looks like your medical identity still hasn't been recognized, try the obvious: "Gosh! It's tough being a *doctor!* That must be the *hospital!*"

4. Wear a white coat or surgical scrubs—but only if you are going to a bar not often frequented by your colleagues. Even though the white coat and scrubs might attract promising material more efficiently, your colleagues will die laughing (there is something to be said for not being *too* obvious), and they will ridicule you for weeks back at the hospital.

That Medical Mystique

Who is it exactly, you lustful would-be doctors ask, who regard a doctor—no matter how slobbish, selfish, and dull—as a catch?

Vast hordes of women, that's who. Lab techs. Dieticians. Ward clerks. X-ray techs. Pharmacists. Secretaries. Nurses of all size, shape, and description. And if you're lucky possibly an administrator, or even (now that med schools have gone co-ed) a fellow physician. And that's just *in* the hospital.

Why is it exactly that these women regard you as a catch? Have you ever heard the saying, "When you see a situation that you cannot understand, look for the financial incentive"?

But remember that you are vulnerable—it's not easy to cope with such large doses of adoration. You've never had much of a social life. You've been too busy trying to get into—and then stay in—medical school. You're an anxious, overworked nerd. Suddenly a gorgeous creature who in your former incarnation wouldn't give you the time of day is bent on meeting, winning, and marrying you. And marriage probably sounds pretty good. You're becoming accustomed to a clean apartment and a well-stocked refrigerator, with delicious food and charming company . . . especially in comparison to your dingy apartment filled with decaying cafeteria food, stacks of old medical journals, and dirty surgical scrubs.

So marriage doesn't sound bad. But you're still not 100 percent sure? This quiz could just save you from investing in an unreturnable engagement ring.

Marriage: Should You or Shouldn't You? Only Your Stockbroker Knows for Sure!

1. **You're thinking about marriage because**
   a. you've been dating four years and you're deeply in love.
   b. she's been nagging you about it.
   c. she says she's pregnant.

2. **Thinking about her meeting your mother makes you**
   a. proud.
   b. anxious.
   c. cringe.

3. **Her favorite activity is**
   a. skiing, tutoring gifted children, playing the violin.
   b. window shopping for an engagement ring.
   c. Out of bed, you aren't too sure.

4. **What you like about her most is**
   a. her intellect, compassion, humor.
   b. She's nice, and she's always available when you call.
   c. She's ready, willing, and able.

5. **She last had to break a date with you because**
   a. she had a sales meeting in New York.
   b. she went to a bridal shower for her *younger* sister.
   c. She's never broken a date. Nothing in her life is more important than you—not her family, her job, her friends, *not even* a Cars concert.

6. **When she reads**
   a. she becomes deeply engrossed.
   b. she moves her lips.
   c. You've never seen her read. You're not sure she can do more than stumble through the back of a cereal box.

7. **She belongs to the following professional organizations:**
   a. Phi Beta Kappa.
   b. Kappa Alpha Theta soriority.
   c. Residents' Wives and Girlfriends' Club.

8. Her single greatest achievement in the last five years has been

   a. publishing her doctoral thesis.

   b. being a varsity cheerleader three years straight.

   c. catching you.

9. The single greatest reason you can think of for marrying is

   a. you love each other.

   b. you like each other.

   c. you can't face another night of hot dogs in a messy, lonely apartment.

Key:

If you answered a to most questions: If you get married, you might stay married.

If you answered b to most questions: If you get married, the chances of staying married through the Reagan administration are minimal. (And he's *not* going to be reelected.) Haven't you wondered why she asks all those questions about the future worth of your M.D. as part of community property?

If you answered c to most questions: If you get married? Well, as they say to the terminal cancer patient, don't buy any long-playing records! Go ahead and get married, if the only choice is between marrying a stranger or a .357 Magnum to the temples. But remember: The only thing worse than being horribly lonely is being horribly lonely and going through a divorce.

The Good, the Bad, and the Ugly: The Women in Mr. Dr.'s Life

The Hometown Honey

Nice girl from back home; they met in high school and married when he was in college. Looked great back in Biloxi, but did not make the transition to the Big City with grace.

   She:

- worked as a secretary to support him through college and medical school.
- packs his lunch every day.
- calls him at work three times a day to see what's up.

   Identifying feature: Continuously pregnant.

The Hometown Honey

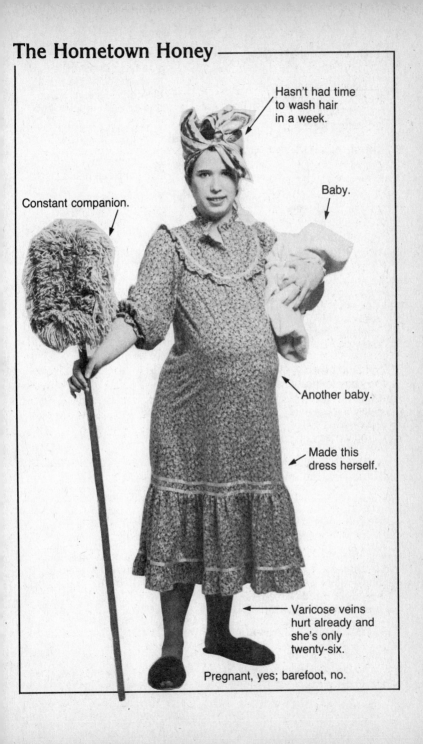

Hasn't had time to wash hair in a week.

Baby.

Constant companion.

Another baby.

Made this dress herself.

Varicose veins hurt already and she's only twenty-six.

Pregnant, yes; barefoot, no.

The Total Nurse

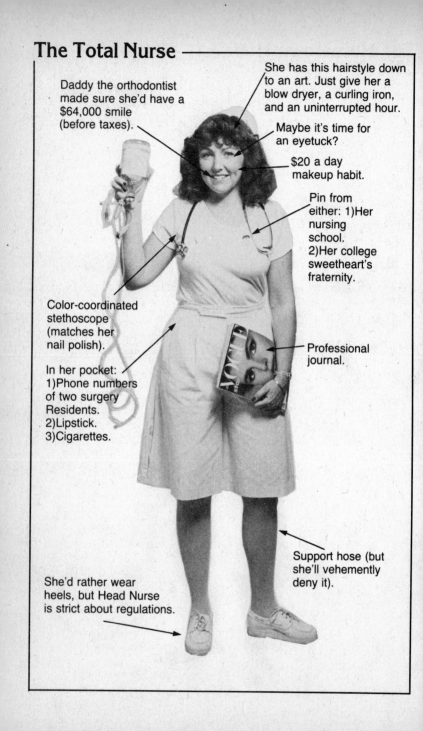

Daddy the orthodontist made sure she'd have a $64,000 smile (before taxes).

She has this hairstyle down to an art. Just give her a blow dryer, a curling iron, and an uninterrupted hour.

Maybe it's time for an eyetuck?

$20 a day makeup habit.

Pin from either: 1)Her nursing school. 2)Her college sweetheart's fraternity.

Color-coordinated stethoscope (matches her nail polish).

In her pocket: 1)Phone numbers of two surgery Residents. 2)Lipstick. 3)Cigarettes.

Professional journal.

Support hose (but she'll vehemently deny it).

She'd rather wear heels, but Head Nurse is strict about regulations.

The Hometown Honey (Cont.)

Clothing: Maternity.

Hobbies: Having babies, cleaning the house.

Topics of conversation: Having babies, cleaning the house.

Most frequent statement: "Honey, you never spend enough time at home."

Favorite Activities:
• Making her own clothes.
• Planning what they'll do with their disposable income, as soon as they get some.

Most common worry: The specter of divorce.

Favorite Magazine: Ladies' Home Journal

Last Book Read: Love's Savage Desire, or anything by Dr. Spock.

Most recent accomplishment: Having Robert, Jr.

Our doctor will probably ditch her for Wife #2 as soon as he gets his M.D., as he becomes more sophisticated and attractive to other women, and as she becomes buried in diapers.

The Total Nurse

A marginally attractive woman who works very hard to look good. Gets up at 5:30 A.M. to put face on, set hair, and make breakfast for whatever Resident spent the night.

Has a terrific figure, courtesy of Dexatrim and diuretics.

Has dated more than 200 Residents, and slept with at least 20. Issues *the ultimatum* after dating a

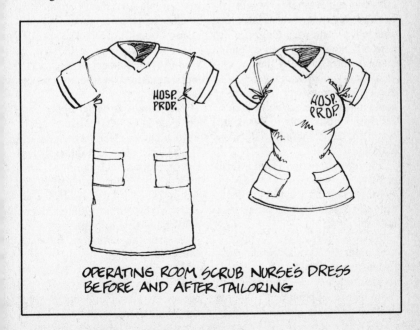

OPERATING ROOM SCRUB NURSE'S DRESS
BEFORE AND AFTER TAILORING

Resident for six months: *Play me or trade me*.

Identifying feature: Always at the hospital watering hole by 5 P.M. Friday at the most accessible, highest-visibility table. Always comes with a girlfriend. Always in separate cars.

Clothing: Uniforms that maximally display the aforementioned figure. Popular items include:

1. translucent T-shirt with hip-gripping culottes.
2. tight see-through white pants with visible bikini underwear, topped by tight white turtlenecks with tiny preppie prints.
3. operating-room scrub dresses that have been drastically tailored

Hobbies: Shopping for clothes, lingerie, makeup, husbands.

Topics of conversation: Hospital gossip—who are the newly divorced surgeons, who's sleeping with whom, and what those new Interns are like—and variations on the theme of how crummy nursing is.

Most frequent statement: "Why don't you come over to dinner? I could throw together some quiche and wine." (Said only to Residents, *never* to techs, administrators, or male nurses.)

Favorite activity: Dating Residents.

Most common worry: The Residents are looking younger (and she's not).

Favorite magazine: Cosmopolitan, naturally; *Vogue* when she's feeling intellectual.

Most recent accomplishment: Head Nurse appointment. No big deal; she'd rather quit.

The Woman Doctor: Type A Nice and Nonthreatening

She isn't very pretty and has no time to maximize the good points she does have. She's gained ten pounds during her internship (doughnuts for dinner will do it!), but hasn't had time to buy clothes that fit.

She's *very* bright and slightly neurotic. She loves being a doctor and works very hard to give good patient care. She's generally cheerful and upbeat, and genuinely *likes* her patients. Despite her exhaustion, she spends extra time with her patients and organizes the Resident-Staff softball games. She occasionally brings in brownies for her team or leans on the attending staff to take a worn-out team out to lunch.

She went to a good women's school—Smith, Holyoke, or Barnard—and majored in Classics or History, then spent a few years working before deciding to become a doctor.

She comes from an upper-middle-class family that expected her to have a career. Her mother has always worked, as an English professor or professional violinist. She's had the obligatory suburban "enriching" experiences—either Foreign Exchange in Guatemala or Outward Bound to Nepal—and she goes with the family to Bermuda every Easter.

Identifying features: Permanent dark circles under eyes with her beeper in status epilepticus—but she's still trying to smile!

The Woman Doctor: Type A — Nice and Nonthreatening

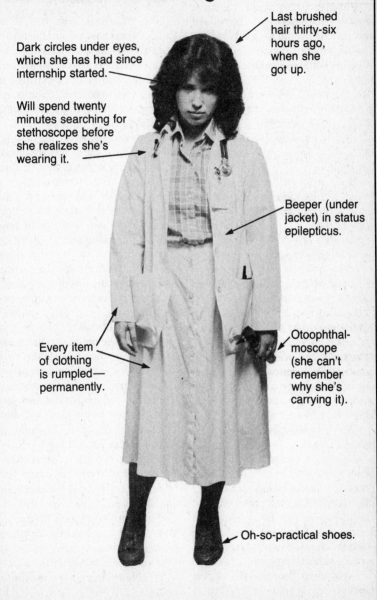

Last brushed hair thirty-six hours ago, when she got up.

Dark circles under eyes, which she has had since internship started.

Will spend twenty minutes searching for stethoscope before she realizes she's wearing it.

Beeper (under jacket) in status epilepticus.

Every item of clothing is rumpled—permanently.

Otoophthal-moscope (she can't remember why she's carrying it).

Oh-so-practical shoes.

Clothing: A mess; looks like she slept in them (she did).

Hobbies: She used to have them—she played viola in college and picked up the art of Nouvelle Cuisine on her Junior Year Abroad. Now she watches *Fantasy Island* reruns.

Topics of conversation: All the great things she and her boyfriend are going to do with their free time—go to foreign films, Indian restaurants, the Cape, skiing—once they get some.

Most frequent statement: "A party? You're kidding. I'd love to, but I'm on call that night. No—go without me."

Favorite activity: Good sex. But don't tell her mother.

Most common worry: How to reconcile being a good doctor with being a good mother.

Favorite magazine: The New England Journal of Medicine

Last book read: Hasn't read recreationally in a year; watches mind-numbing TV reruns when she's tired. When she's really peppy, she'll do aerobics to old tapes of *The Prairie Home Companion*.

Most recent accomplishment: She brought a sixty-year-old man through a massive myocardial infarction, complicated by heart failure, hypotension, cardiogenic shock, cardiac arrhythmias, and pneumonia for *six weeks* in the Intensive Care Unit—and *shook his hand* as he **walked out** the door. (He later wrote a sweet letter to her parents, saying, "Your darling daughter the doctor must gives you *nachis* every day.")

The Woman Doctor: Type B The Killer Female

She graduated from M.I.T. or Duke, where she published madly as an undergraduate. She has at least one advanced degree in addition to her M.D., and is board-certified in at least two specialties. She is interested in Hematology/Oncology, and she plans to be chairman of a good department before she's forty. At thirty-five, she's already turned down offers from lesser departments.

She enjoys making Residents quiver and full professors acutely anxious with her displays of brilliance and erudition. She chews up the uninformed and the slow, and spits them out. She speaks in complete, grammatical sentences at top speed, and never hesitates or gropes for words. She *never* prefaces statements with "I think" or "It seems to me"; rather she predicates her every hopelessly complex sentence with *"Obviously* the problem here is" or "It *should* be clear to you all that . . ."

She's divorced, but does not talk about it. She now dates only successful department chairmen of macho specialties. Rumor has it she pays alimony to her ex, a pediatrician in the boonies.

Identifying feature: Always engaged in a goal-directed activity.

Clothing: Absolutely utilitarian. Has twenty multiseason, interchangeable blouses and skirts and four pairs of sensible shoes.

Hobbies: Does not waste time on hobbies.

The Woman Doctor: Type B — The Killer Female

"What do you *mean* you just don't know?"

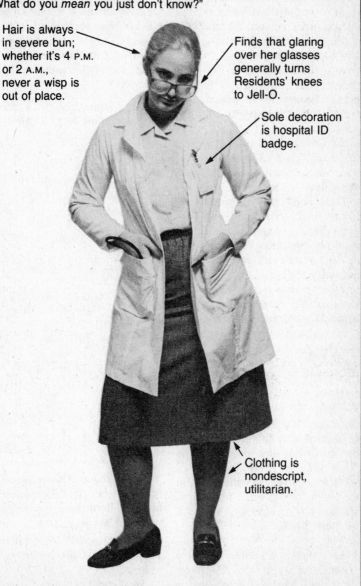

Hair is always in severe bun; whether it's 4 P.M. or 2 A.M., never a wisp is out of place.

Finds that glaring over her glasses generally turns Residents' knees to Jell-O.

Sole decoration is hospital ID badge.

Clothing is nondescript, utilitarian.

Topics of conversation: Journal articles, Basic Pathophysiology, statistical analysis of research data.

Most frequent statement: "What do you *mean* you don't know?"

Favorite activity: Castrating Residents on rounds.

Most common worry: Her most recent NIH grant won't be approved, because it's too complex for the NIH review board to fully understand.

Favorite magazines: Subscribes to 6 + professional journals; reads, understands, and quotes from them every day.

Last book read: Grossman's *Cardiac Catheterization and Angiography.* In one night. And picked up three mistakes. Which she, of course, reported to Dr. Grossman himself.

Most recent accomplishment: Rounded her remarkable score of Resident withdrawals to an even 10.

The Ward Clerk with More Bust Than Brains

She's so incredibly simple that she finds filing and sorting a real challenge. She likes the excitement of hospital work (it's just like TV!), but never has any idea of what's going on. She's always surprised when a massively ill patient dies in the night. "Oh, that nice Mr. Krebs! He didn't even *look* sick, except for all those tubes in his nose!"

She:

- dates Medical Students (whom she flatters at work by calling them "doctor" when everyone else is calling them "stupid").

- is always available on short notice to spend the night in the on-call room (but doesn't understand why her nickname is Room Service).
- is not into women's liberation.
- works only to kill time before marriage and babies.
- will marry a lab tech or orderly at thirty.

Identifying feature: Feminine giggles coming from a male Resident's on-call room.

Clothing: Slit skirts up to the waist; plunging blouses down to the waist. She is always trendy: miniskirts, spangled leg warmers, sweat shirt dresses in purple and black, and a wardrobe of other ensembles better suited to a nightclub than a hospital.

Hobbies: Loves to disco and do 'ludes (is not bright enough to realize that her dates take her to out-of-the-way places where they won't be seen).

Topics of conversation:
- Where to disco and with whom.
- Who Mick Jagger is dating.
- Elizabeth Taylor's weight problem.
- Michael Landon's rocky marriage.
- In other words, anything from the *National Enquirer.*

Most frequent statement: "The vesicles from my last episode are healed. Really—I promise you won't get herpes."

Favorite activity: Watching *Real People, That's Incredible,* or any soap.

Most common worries:
- Do I have a date for Saturday?

The Ward Clerk with More Bust Than Brains

"Let's go Disco!"

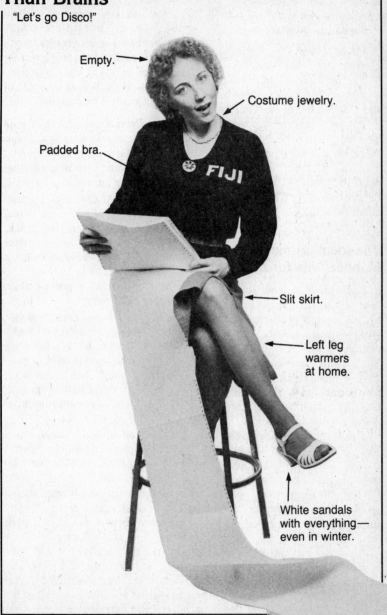

Empty.

Costume jewelry.

Padded bra.

FIJI

Slit skirt.

Left leg warmers at home.

White sandals with everything— even in winter.

- Will Melba on *General Hospital* tell Ned it's not his baby?
- Is Princess Di secretly miserable?
- Maybe I'm pregnant?

Favorite magazine: Reads the captions in *People*.

Last book read: Part of the Monarch notes for *Hamlet* right before she dropped out of eleventh grade.

Most recent accomplishment: She was the principal vector for an in-house herpes epidemic that included 5 medical students, 6 surgery residents, 4 Nurses, 11 Ward Clerks, 2 internists, and the Chairman of Psychiatry's wife.

The Ideal Girlfriend/ Fiancée/Wife for a Doctor

She's pretty, but not so stunning that he's worried she'll leave him. She is always well-groomed and wears conspicuously expensive clothing in wool, cashmere, or silk. She's always neat and well put together without looking as if she spent all morning at it (and she wears makeup so well he's convinced she doesn't wear any at all).

She's *not* in medicine! She's in some glamorous field—publishing, the arts, academics—that keeps her busy but *never* keeps her from taking time off for him. She will preferably inherit money, so her zilch future earning power doesn't matter.

She has nice, interesting friends who are thrilled to meet a real doctor—even if he's just a Dermatologist—and will love hearing stories about his exciting medical career—

even if his stories are borrowed or fictitious.

She can talk animatedly about many subjects, but she doesn't object when he and his cronies launch into subjects that hold no interest for her, such as "Why the department chairman is such a schmuck," or "My ten greatest cases as an intern."

Identifying feature: She is seen at stuffy formal departmental parties charming the department chairman, whom everyone else is too intimidated to even *approach*.

Clothing: Always classic, neat, and attractive.

For work—anything from Talbot's.

For play—anything from L. L. Bean's.

For dress-up—anything from Bergdorf's or Saks.

Hobbies: Plays all racquet sports well enough to be a decent mixed-doubles partner. Is cheerful while playing, works hard to win but *never* curses or pouts when beaten. She swims seriously to keep in (terrific) shape. She likes to collect antiques but does not insist that he accompany her on antiquing jaunts—she's just as happy to go with mother.

Topics of conversation: She's the consummate mixer. She talks about whatever other people want to talk about, and asks very interested questions about them and their work. If pressed, she will briefly discuss her work or family, but will never bore or intimidate. She *never* discusses her husband's cases, even though he tells her everything. She *never* discusses particulars of her

The Ideal Girlfriend/Fiancée/Wife

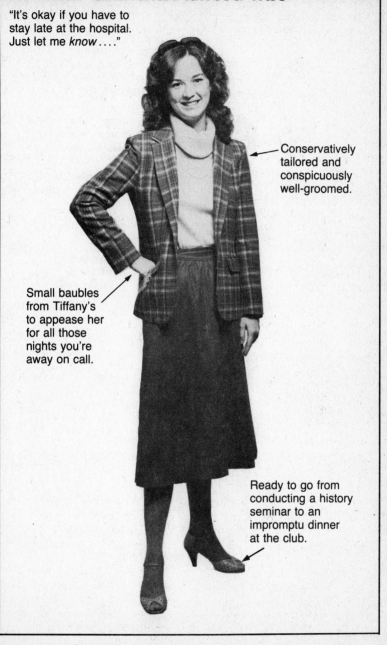

"It's okay if you have to stay late at the hospital. Just let me *know*...."

Conservatively tailored and conspicuously well-groomed.

Small baubles from Tiffany's to appease her for all those nights you're away on call.

Ready to go from conducting a history seminar to an impromptu dinner at the club.

The Ideal Girlfriend/Fiancée/Wife

"Just a suggestion, honey. Greece would be okay, too."

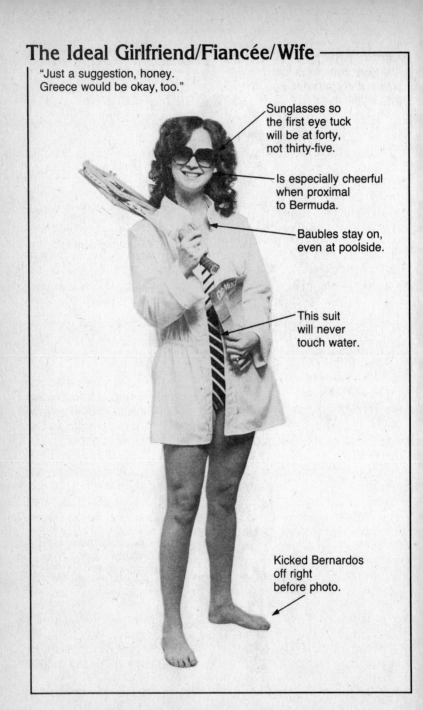

Sunglasses so the first eye tuck will be at forty, not thirty-five.

Is especially cheerful when proximal to Bermuda.

Baubles stay on, even at poolside.

This suit will never touch water.

Kicked Bernardos off right before photo.

husband's practice and dismisses any nosy questions with "Oh, everything's fine. And how's *your* husband's business?"

Favorite activities:

- going to glittery nightspots and meeting a few major and a couple of minor celebrities.
- skiing at Saint Moritz for Christmas.
- feeding the ducks at the local town pond.
- choosing a Saint Bernard puppy for her niece.
- attending big family Thanksgiving gatherings.

Most common worries:

- Can we get tickets to *Cats*?
- Are Rossignols better than Olins?
- Will I ever learn to do fellatio right?

Favorite magazines: Vogue. The New Yorker. Savvy (but wouldn't be caught dead reading it).

Last book read: Something by Jane Austen.

Most recent accomplishment: One of the following:

- Teaching the entire fifth grade at the Scarsdale Fox Meadow Elementary School to sing a significant chunk of Handel's *Messiah,* or
- Publishing her doctoral thesis in *Annals of Archaeology,* or
- Getting an audition with the Joffrey Ballet, or
- Successfully organizing a Planned Parenthood fund-raiser at the Aquarium.

Profiles in Tenacity: How to Meet and Marry a Doctor

Remember Willie Sutton's admonition!

When he was asked why he robbed banks, he said, "Because that's where the money is."

Ergo: If you want to meet and marry a doctor, *go to the hospital.* Definitely don't waste your time in bars or health clubs, where you have to spend twenty minutes talking to guys before you discover that they aren't even gainfully employed.

Think of the Hospital as a Giant Singles' Supermarket

The doctors are even uniformed, labeled, and color-coded according to type—the better to focus your efforts on the upper-echelon staff in the high-paying specialties!

Go to the hospital

You can go as a patient. This works better in the movies than in real life. A Hollywood plot staple is the stunningly beautiful woman who is dying from a disease that makes her legs longer, her cheekbones more pronounced, and her bust bigger. (I've looked—this disease is *not* in the textbooks.) Of course, all the interns fall passionately in love with her, and a tearjerker wedding ceremony is performed in her laminar-flow isolation room.

In reality, however, it's tough to look decent—let alone beautiful—when you are ill. Remember the last time you had the flu? Swollen eyes, runny nose, flushed face? Real seductive. Can you imagine the end of *Love Story* with a nasogastric tube up Ali MacGraw's nose?

Ethical doctors don't date patients, anyway.

You can go to medical school. Attending medical school to marry a doctor is like climbing Mount Everest to get some fresh mountain air.

You can be a nurse. An arduous but effective route, as many happily married and now retired nurses will attest. Although nursing is not as hard to get into as medical school, actually *being* a nurse is tedious, difficult, and poorly paid.

None of these options sounds appealing, we know. That's why you need to try to *work in the hospital*—in a nonmedical job. You want a job that is: *1. High-visibility:* i.e., working with doctors every day in an office. *Not* supervising housekeeping. And *don't* get stuck in the insurance typing pool.

2. Not strenuous: So you have plenty of time to chat, to fix your makeup and hair, and so you can wear foot-deforming high heels every day to work.

Pay is unimportant; volunteer if you have to. What could be cuter than you in a pink volunteer smock, a little ray of sunshine wheeling candy and flowers around to the patients?

Just being *in* the hospital isn't enough, of course; you must aggressively *identify* and *track* your quarry. *Read name tags!* Not every man in a white coat is a doctor; be wary of handsome pharmacists, respiratory therapists, social workers, and male nurses.

Smile at *every* Resident and call him by name. He may be happily married, but he might well have doctor friends who aren't. Besides, it makes your single-minded pursuit less obvious if you happily chat with married doctors and women doctors. Your unwitting single prey will relax.

Once you have cut your Resident out from the herd (pick a lonely, or funny-looking, or otherwise not-so-attractive one; the handsomest Resident in the hospital already has 500 women in hot pursuit), don't immediately pounce. Move slowly but surely (he *doesn't* need to meet your folks on the third date).

1. Invite him for a home-cooked meal.
2. Expect him to be late/forget entirely.
3. Be sweet about it when he is late/forgets entirely.
4. Be persistent in rescheduling dates.

Don't be intimidated by the professional women in the hospital. Although the women doctors and nurses have more in common with him, and so have more shared topics of conversation, they can be threatening. You have the advantage; you have the time, energy, and inclination to dress well and *to look ter-*

rific every day. Women doctors are too tired and busy to spend time on personal beauty, and nurses are trapped in uniforms that would make Cheryl Tiegs look like the Goodyear Blimp. Besides, the nurses and doctors are too busy coping with work, while *you* have time on your hands.

The Right Approach: The Very Best High-profile Jobs in the Hospital

1. The Very Best Job: Secretary to the Department Chairman. You'll spend all day working with Residents and staff. You're in a position of power and can grant favors to friends—a peek at their secret files, a rescheduled appointment, a gauge of the chairman's mood that day.

2. Operating-room Scheduling Secretary: You will have every surgeon in town on his knees to you, so you will preferentially schedule his cases. Again, you are in a position to dispense favors.

3. Check-out at the Hospital Cafeteria: A high-profile but low-class job. Therefore, you must place a copy of Proust's *Remembrance of Things Past* or perhaps *Greek Art Treasures* next to your cash register to counteract the reflex feeling that you are not bright. Great job because of frequent, repeated exposure to Residents (who eat breakfast, lunch, dinner, and midnight snack in hospital), especially late at night when they are lonely and bored; you can also sneak free food to Residents, who are perpetually broke and hungry.

How to Make Conversation with a Resident

Okay, so you look terrific, and he's seen you around the hospital. Now you want to start a conversation. Residents are unable to talk about the usual everyday chatter; they do not read the newspapers or watch the news, so they don't know about the blizzard in Atlanta, the U.S.-Japan trade agreements, or what happened to Hinckley. They may keep up on professional sports, but chances are you don't. They have no hobbies—except for going home to sleep and fight roaches—and few outside interests. You can certainly give politics and culture and the weather a try, but when all else fails, there are two sure-fire conversation staples guaranteed to spark a Resident's interest:

1. Their patients. Surgical triumphs. Medical disasters. Strange family arrangements. Bizarre self-treatments. Residents like to talk about their patients, especially when the Resident made a difficult diagnosis or successful treatment. (*Tip:* Don't bring up disasters. Residents have to talk about their disasters much more than they would prefer to.)

2. Their residency. Residents are generally unhappy with their residency; they think that they are in the wrong specialty or that they would have been happier at a different hospital.

To make the conversation work, however, you must talk about these subjects as though they truly interest you. And never, but never, attempt

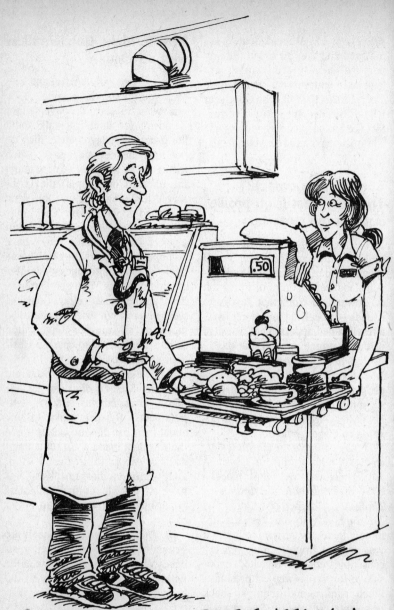

THE VERY BEST HIGH PROFILE JOBS IN THE HOSPITAL (TO MEET AND MARRY A DOCTOR)

to introduce such topics of conversation as:

- The complications of your mother's gall-bladder surgery
- Why you hate your hair color
- How much you want to be married

The average Resident, who never had manners *before* residency, is now completely devoid of social graces and will bolt from the room, without explanation, when these topics come up.

Just remember: With a lot of effort, a little luck, and intense perseverance, you, too, can land a doctor of your very own!

The Social Life of Women Doctors

The only person trying to railroad *you* into marriage is your mother.

It is difficult to build a sparkling social life from the truly dismal raw material on your plate. During the course of a typical surgery rotation workday at a Veterans Administration Hospital, you might meet:

- two married middle-aged surgeons, both interested in a fling.
- two shakily married surgery Residents, too tired to think about fooling around.
- one gay surgery Resident.
- one single surgery Resident, with 32 nurses in hot pursuit.
- a busboy.
- an elevator operator.

- twenty-seven veterans in various stages of renal failure, hepatic encephalopathy, cardiac decompensation, alcoholic dementia, heroin withdrawal, and septic shock.

But what about outside the hospital?

Is it really so much to ask for, an attractive, pleasant, well-educated man who is secure enough to accept your social status and earning capacity? Maybe. Maybe not.

You may actually find that man. But odds are that he will be one of three things: 1) gay, 2) married, or 3) dating your best friend.

So much for your best friend.

Ms. Doctor's Husbands and Boyfriends

As a group, they are:

- very smart
- very successful
- and very well-educated, not to mention
- quite ambitious
- very self-assured
- ten years older than their wives

Mostly in medicine, they are either in the "macho" fields like Thoracic Surgery, Cardiology, Emergency Medicine, or in the fields that make minimal demands (comparatively) on their time—the life-style fields like Radiology, Pathology, Anesthesiology, Ophthalmology.

Those who aren't in medicine are attorneys, tenured professors, or entrepreneurial geniuses.

Social Life of Women Doctors

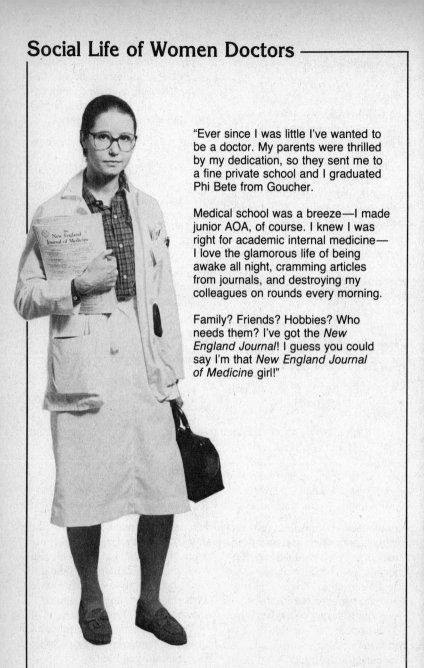

"Ever since I was little I've wanted to be a doctor. My parents were thrilled by my dedication, so they sent me to a fine private school and I graduated Phi Bete from Goucher.

Medical school was a breeze—I made junior AOA, of course. I knew I was right for academic internal medicine—I love the glamorous life of being awake all night, cramming articles from journals, and destroying my colleagues on rounds every morning.

Family? Friends? Hobbies? Who needs them? I've got the *New England Journal*! I guess you could say I'm that *New England Journal of Medicine* girl!"

Profile of the Ideal Husband for a Doctor

Identifying feature:

* radiates self-confidence.
* is self-sufficient, a great cook, and good at housework.

Clothing: Shabby academic (i.e., well-worn Brooks Brothers with leather-patched elbows on the good Harris Tweed jacket).

Hobbies: Bird-watching, opera.

Topics of conversation: Everything—as long as his conversation partner is well-informed and succinct.

Most frequent statement: "I read an article about that recently, and I think..."

Most common worry: Will his outside interests distract him from achieving in his chosen career? (Is not in the slightest bit worried that his wife may earn more than he does, and is quite willing to cheerfully spend whatever she makes.)

Favorite activities:

* Bearbaiting Pavlovian liberals
* Squash
* Erotic journals, i.e., *Playboy*

Magazine: Used to read *Harper's* but quit when it became intellectually sloppy; now reads *The Atlantic Monthly*. Has read *The New Yorker* since high school but only recently has discovered that its fiction is as good as the book excerpts.

Last book read: The Power Broker by Robert Caro—he is one of the few people in America to have read the entire 1,200-page tome. Before that, Barbara Tuchman's *A Distant Mirror*—again, the entire twenty-pound thing.

Most recent accomplishment: Found, after a long search, an excellent, convenient day-care center for their three-year-old son. Doesn't mind ferrying the tyke back and forth, either—"After all, honey, my hours are more predictable than yours."

Five Warning Signs of MOR Syndrome; or, Marriage on the Rocks

1. Your spouse asks you to put a numerical value on your future earnings, "just out of curiosity."

2. S/He starts talking about divorced sister Sarah, who married a gastroenterologist but didn't realize what a jerk he was until they were married for six months. You've been married six months.

3. Your mother-in-law calls and says, "Oh, you still live there?"

4. S/He doesn't even complain when you call to say you'll be home late, again.

5. You run into each other at a notorious singles' bar. You aren't with a group of friends, and neither is s/he.

Profile of the Ideal Husband for a Doctor

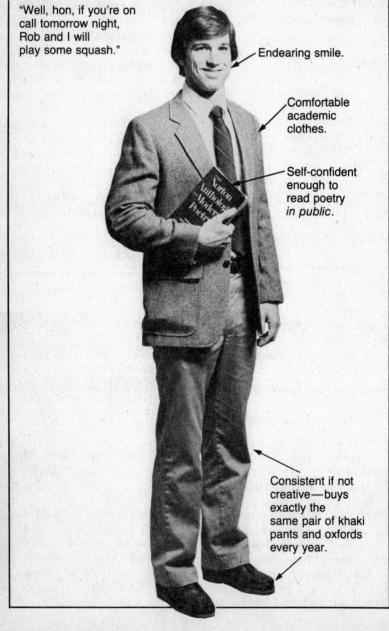

"Well, hon, if you're on call tomorrow night, Rob and I will play some squash."

Endearing smile.

Comfortable academic clothes.

Self-confident enough to read poetry *in public*.

Consistent if not creative—buys exactly the same pair of khaki pants and oxfords every year.

Doctors' Spare-time Activities; or, How to Fill Up Those Yawning Empty Twenty Minutes of Unscheduled Activity Every Day

a. Sleep.

b. Nap.

c. Doze.

d. Call home and see if your kids recognize your voice.

e. See how many bills have fallen behind the refrigerator. Stack them neatly. Put them back behind the refrigerator.

f. Take the car to the garage to get those bizarre noises and billowing black smoke fixed, only to have the mechanic say, "If this was a horse I'd shoot it and put it out of its misery."

g. Go to the grocery and stock up on frozen dinners.

h. Call your parents. Tell them you're still alive.

What Do Medical Students/Doctors Do Together on a Night Off?

1. Get far, far away from each other. (Would you do *anything* with a co-worker you just ate, worked, and slept with for thirty-six hours?)

2. Go out and get falling-down drunk together. Rehash hospital politics.

3. Discuss all the reasons it was foolish to go into Surgery/Medicine/Pediatrics.

4. Make dates to play squash/tennis/racquetball. They will inevitably be broken at the last minute because you can't get out of hospital.

5. Make dates to go out with co-workers and spouses. One, both, or all four of you break it at the last minute because you can't get out of the hospital.

6. Actually manage to get a group together for the movies, but everyone falls asleep. After movie, go for coffee and try to piece together the movie's plot.

What Do Medical Students Do In their Spare Time?

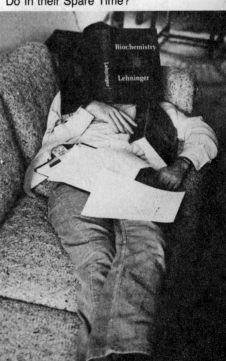

Life on the Outside: Apartment Dwelling
The Medical Student's Apartment—
usually a dormitory room or a one-room efficiency

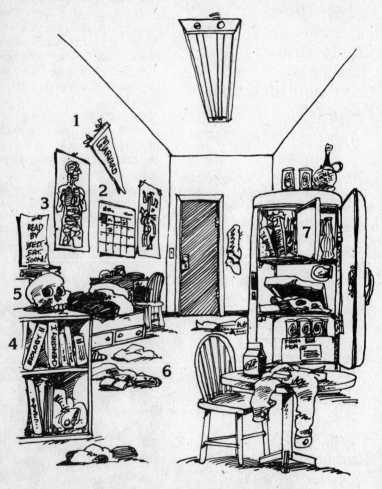

1. College pennant (from a better school than you actually went to)
2. Overcrowded calendar of test/exam/paper due-dates
3. Items to impress dates—Complex Biochemical Pathway chart
                         Complex Gross Anatomy Poster
4. College Chemistry, Biology, and Physics (a reminder of when life was simple and work was easy)
5. Skull from Gross Anatomy (also to impress dates)
6. Wardrobe items
7. Foodstuffs

The Resident's Apartment—a dark, one-bedroom apartment near the hospital (usually on the bad side of town)

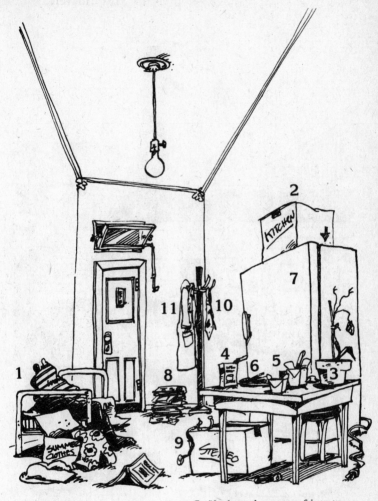

1. Unmade bed
2. Unpacked packing boxes
3. One dead plant
4. Instant breakfast
5. Antique Chinese food cartons
6. Two forks and one plate, property of Doherty County General Hospital
7. Unplugged, empty refrigerator
8. Back issues of *The New England Journal*— unread, of course
9. Broken stethoscope
10. Dirty ties
11. Formerly-white coats

The Real Doctor's Apartment—stereotypically plush, a huge split-level with floor-to-ceiling windows and winding staircase

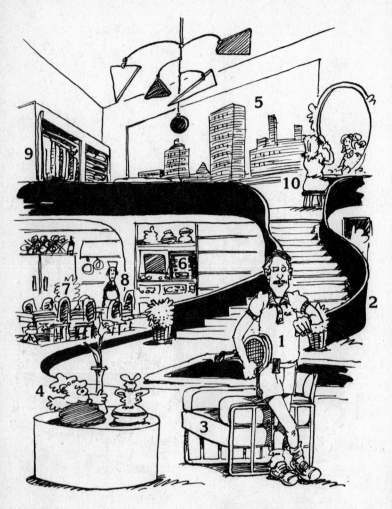

1. Doctor
2. Teak banisters
3. beige upholstery
4. Genuine Pre-Columbian art
5. Spectacular skyline view
6. State-of-the-art stereo
7. Fresh flowers—daily
8. Maid
9. Brooks Brothers' best
10. Wife

Real Doctors Don't Eat Quiche

What do they eat?

Medical Students live on a solid diet of humble pie, fed to them day after grueling day by Residents and staff.

Residents are more nutritionally sophisticated; they make sure to get the U.S. minimum daily requirement of each of the four basic food groups:

1. *Nicotine:* They are careful to smoke at least three cigarettes between every surgical case.
2. *Caffeine:* By residency this action is a reflex. Every time they sit down, they drink a cup of coffee, which helps to keep them conscious (if not alert and oriented).
3. *Carbohydrates:* Residents get the required load of refined white sugar by eating a dessert with every meal—including breakfast and midnight snack—for "extra energy."
4. *Food preservatives:* They eat all meals in the hospital cafeteria, where food preservatives sprinkled with artificial coloring is the main ingredient of every dish.

Real Doctors are nutritionally finicky and will eat only:

1. Haute cuisine
2. Nouvelle Cuisine
3. Good Chinese or Thai food

Real Doctors go to the hospital cafeteria only for coffee, and then rarely (the secretary usually runs out to the corner deli for it).

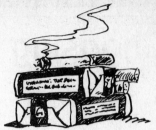

NICOTINE

CAFFEINE

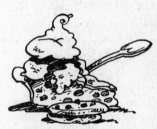

CARBOHYDRATES

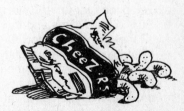

FOOD PRESERVATIVES

CHAPTER 7

Choosing a Specialty

So you've survived medical school—but that's only the first step. What about a specialty? Perhaps you've thought, as you expertly sliced up turkey for the kids' sandwiches, that you'd be a great Surgeon? Or maybe, as you counseled yet another friend embroiled in a dying love affair, that you could be a Psychiatrist?

All those specialties. How do you pick the one that's right for you? And once you make your choice, what will your life be like? How can you find out?

You could throw the next decade of your life away training to be a General Surgeon only to discover that you'd be a better and happier Dermatologist.

Or you could take the *Minnesota Multi-phasic Specialty Inventory*.

The Minnesota Multi-phasic Specialty Inventory

1. **The sight of blood**
   a. makes you queasy.
   b. quickens your pulse and gives you an instant erection.
   c. makes you immediately think about the impact of aspirin on platelet aggregation and the overall incidence of cerebral thromboembolic phenomenon.

2. **You witness a car accident in the street.**
   a. Telephone for an ambulance.
   b. Run to the victims and try to take charge, announcing, "Out of the way! I know *CPA!*" Attempt to direct everything, from resuscitation of the injured to mechanical disengagement of the impacted autos.
   c. Run to the victims and point out to the rapidly expiring one that his chances for survival would have been 56 percent greater had he been wearing his seatbelt at the time of impact.

3. **Your beeper goes off at 3 A.M. You**
   a. ignore it and go back to sleep, knowing that if it's really important, they'll call back.
   b. jump into the clothes you keep by the bedside (or perhaps you sleep fully clothed, to be ready for this), leap into your car, and drive to the hospital, quivering with anticipation over the new diagnostic and therapeutic challenges that now await you.
   c. call in and ascertain that the doctor in charge can handle the situation until the morning. Then, stay up all night reading about the problem so you'll look brilliant in the morning.

4. **When thinking about your identity, you would rank yourself as**
   a. parent first, then spouse, American, Republican, doctor.
   b. You never think about psychobabble crap like that.
   c. Doctor. Doctor. Doctor.

5. **When you talk about "the journal" you are referring to:**
   a. *The Wall Street,* of course.
   b. *Car & Driver. Hustler.*
   c. *The New England.*

6. **You attribute your Pac-Man skill to:**
   a. the hours and quarters you've spent playing.
   b. your incredible hand-eye coordination and manual dexterity.
   c. your intellectual capacity to outthink the game.

7. **When your car doesn't work you**
   a. take it to the garage.
   b. decide that you are mechanically adept enough to figure out what's wrong, tinker with it for an afternoon, exacerbate the problem, get angry and vow to never buy a foreign car again, and bellow at the wife to get the damned thing fixed.
   c. buy three handbooks on repairs, read them every night for three nights, construct a vast differential diagnosis for the problem accompanied by meticulous charts and diagrams, but never actually get around to doing anything about the car's problem.

8. If you ran for the elevator and the door was just closing
a. you would stick your hand in the door.
b. you'd stick your foot or head in the door.
c. you'd curse the fates and run up six flights.

9. The most important part of your body is
a. your privates.
b. your hands.
c. the part of your brain capable of memorizing Organic Chemistry.

10. Your brother tells you he is gay. You.
a. sit down and discuss this with him.
b. punch him in the face and call him a fairy.
c. give him six papers on Kaposi's sarcoma and tell him you've always thought that basic biomedical science research was more interesting and a lot safer than sexual adventuring.

Key:

If you answered a to most questions: You are a normal person. You are well-suited to a wide variety of pleasant specialties in medicine that will give you time to raise a family and read the newspaper. Go to Part Two and find out whether you're best suited to Dermatology, Neuroradiology, Blood Bank Pathology, Oculoplastics, or some other obscure but nonstrenuous specialty.

If you answered b to most questions: You're going to be a great Surgeon—one of the world's best. But, of course, you already *knew* that. You have qualities essential to the practice of surgery: extra-large ego, the desire to take charge even when you're not sure what you're taking charge *of,* the inability to self-doubt (which will help when things get rough in the Operating Room), a fundamental love for medicine (which will keep you going despite complete exhaustion), a Good Old Boy Mentality (which will help you get along with your colleagues), and an incredible paranoia about damage to your hands.

If you answered c to most questions: You are perfectly suited for Academic Medicine. You love *facts,* not the application of facts. You'd much rather read about diseases than have to talk with someone who has one. Your absolutely favorite activity is demonstrating how much you know about the topic at hand, whether it's medical, political, or philosophical; you are a star at academic one-up-manship. You are, at this moment, looking for the grading scale to make sure that, once again, you have answered every question on an examination correctly.

Quiz: The Shoes of the Specialist
Match the shoe with its wearer's specialty.

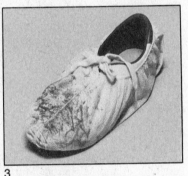

1

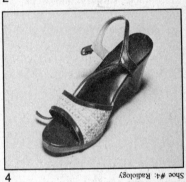

2

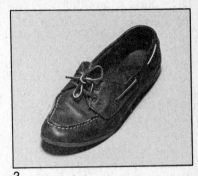

3

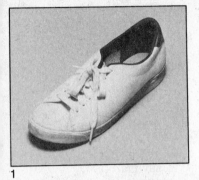

4

Shoe #1: Internal medicine
Shoe #2: Pediatrics
Shoe #3: Surgery
Shoe #4: Radiology

The Truth About the Specialties; or, Television Versus Reality

Forensic pathologists on television traipse around the fashionable nightspots of L.A. picking up women half their age in the routine course of the workday.

Forensic pathologists in real life spend most of the day in the basement of the hospital with fragments of the barely recognizable remains of the victims of the local Knife & Gun Club. For fun, they expose themselves to extremely infectious bacteria, which killed the patients on whom they are performing the autopsies.

General surgeons on television spend hours in the hospital cafeteria chatting about Monica having Alan's baby, only it wasn't really Alan's but someone else's, and the true father doesn't know it, but his *wife* does. . . .

General surgeons in real life gossip, but only intraoperatively, and then usually it involves slander of other surgeons' professional ineptitude and fouled-up cases. General Surgeons *never* sit down to eat lunch; usually they don't even *eat* lunch.

Family practitioners on television make house calls, perform cardiothoracic surgery one week and emergency psychotherapy the next, and are universally loved by all their patients.

Family practitioners in real life are worried about *getting* patients.

But Ten Years Later... Will You Be Employed?

It's wise to train in a specialty that offers at least a chance of employment, so choose your field accordingly:

1. High-paying, pleasant fields that are already overcrowded:
Ear, Nose, Throat (Otolaryngology)
Ophthalmology
Dermatology
Radiology
Plastic Surgery

2. High-paying, not particularly pleasant fields that are also filled:
General Surgery

Obstetrics and Gynecology
Neurosurgery
Gastroenterology

3. High-paying work with good job security but EXTREMELY boring:
Anesthesiology

4. High-paying work with good job security but quite unpleasant:
Pathology

5. Excellent job security but pays poorly:
Psychiatry
Family Practice

6. Only for the anal compulsive:
Academic Medicine and Surgery

Selecting a Specialty Right for You

Those of you who discovered in Part One of the Minnesota Multiphasic Specialty Inventory that both Academic Medicine and Surgery were much too intense, don't lose faith. It's all right that you have run-of-the-mill, mediocre priorities, and would rather be at your daughter's sixth birthday party than mucking around in the Operating Room with some old geezer's hemorrhaging bowel, or would rather be reading Hedrick Smith's *The Russians* than Spaet's *Atherosclerosis in Primates*. If you're willing to tolerate the scorn of the medicine and surgery doctors, it's time for you to pick a laid-back specialty.

Anesthesia

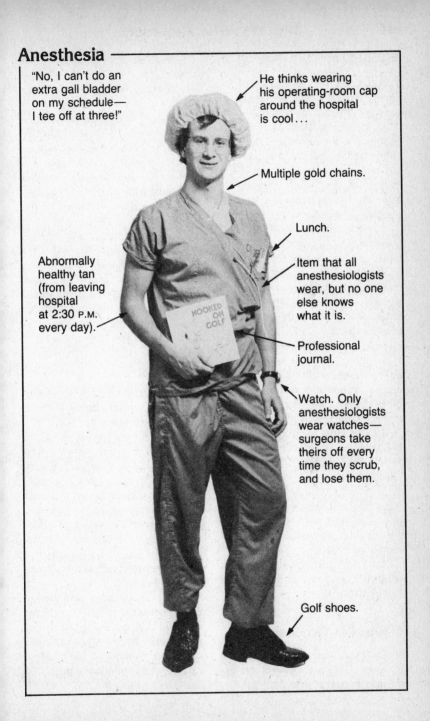

"No, I can't do an extra gall bladder on my schedule— I tee off at three!"

He thinks wearing his operating-room cap around the hospital is cool...

Multiple gold chains.

Lunch.

Item that all anesthesiologists wear, but no one else knows what it is.

Abnormally healthy tan (from leaving hospital at 2:30 P.M. every day).

HOOKED ON GOLF

Professional journal.

Watch. Only anesthesiologists wear watches— surgeons take theirs off every time they scrub, and lose them.

Golf shoes.

Anesthesia

Anesthesiology is the art of inducing unconsciousness in patients, so that surgeons may forcibly restructure their anatomies. Anesthesiology is without a doubt a dull specialty, and the people attracted to it are not especially dynamic. Contrary to public belief, they do do more than just talk to you to put you to sleep—some actually use drugs.

Anesthesiology is 99 percent boredom and 1 percent panic (the panic occurs when the surgeon wakes up the anesthesiologist, who is dozing over the latest issue of *Field & Stream,* and says, "Hey, Joe—I think you attached the heart-lung machine backwards!").

Consider Anesthesia if:

1. People you chat with at cocktail parties get a glazed look in their eyes and suddenly need to get another drink (even though they are already holding full glasses).

2. The most exciting thing that happened on your last vacation was getting stuck in a traffic jam outside Disney World.

3. Your favorite hobby is assembling difficult jigsaw puzzles, especially puzzles that, when completed, represent scrambled jigsaw-puzzle pieces.

4. Your best encounters with people have been when they are sound asleep.

Obstetrics/Gynecology

Can you answer *yes* to these questions? If so, you will be extremely happy in Ob/Gyn.

1. Do you enjoy seeing women in pain?

2. Do you enjoy giving women pain?

3. Are you capable of pontificating about the miracle of birth as you sit between the legs of a hysterical, screaming, just-about-to-deliver mother as gushes of blood and other stuff spray you?

4. Are you not disturbed by the idea of rolling out of bed every third night at age fifty to drive to the hospital through freezing snows?

5. Does the idea of spending your day chatting about painful, irregular menses; foul vaginal discharges; itchy crotches; and highly infectious sexually transmitted diseases actually appeal to you?

Pediatrics

Do you love children? Do you love them when they vomit on you? When they hit you? When they lose their diaper contents on your formerly nice white coat? When they scream, "I hate you, Mr. Doctor!" so loudly that every mother and child in your waiting room is thrown into a panic? How do you feel about chasing a tyke down a hospital corridor as he wails, "Help! Help! The doctor's hurting me!" as you sheepishly jog behind?

You'll be a terrific pediatrician if you answer *yes* to these questions:

1. Do you prefer to wear polyester, drip-dry, no-stain clothing?

2. Is the sound of six children wailing simultaneously music to your ears?

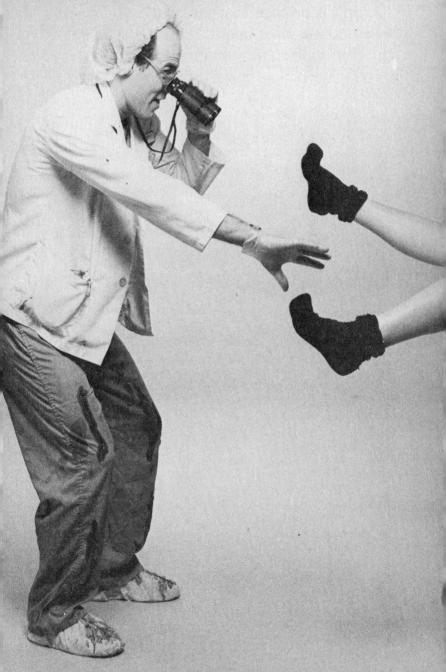

Pediatrics
Wouldn't it be nice to once, just once, be able to listen to a kid's heartbeat without having to first demonstrate on yourself?

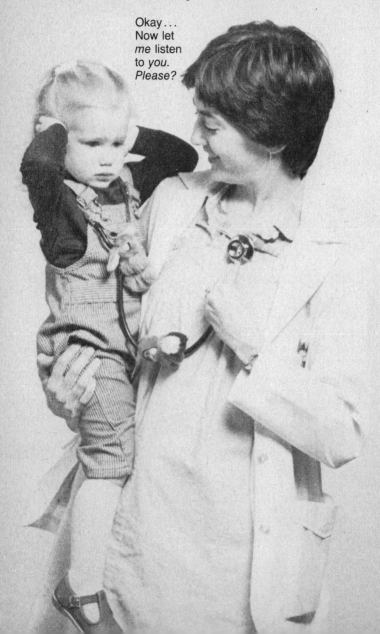

Psychiatry: Close Encounters with Disturbed Minds

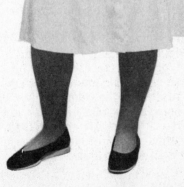

"Can you tell me more about that?"

Natural hair.

Chain-smokes.

Funky organic clothes.

Never a white coat.

(Yes, that's a banana in her pocket... but she's a psychiatrist, after all.)

3. Are you comfortable with the fact that 90 percent of the patients in your waiting room devoutly wish that you would die before their scheduled appointments?

Psychiatry

The world needs more psychiatrists, but few people are signing up for the job. It's not lucrative. It's not glamorous. Your average patient is *not* some lithe young starlet, and you must graciously put up with gratuitous jokes from lay people:

Q. How many psychiatrists does it take to change a light bulb?

A. Only one, but the light bulb has to really *want* to be changed.

Are you neurotic enough to be a psychiatrist? This quiz will tell:

1. **Your wife screams at you, "I hate you and I'm leaving you!" You reply:**
   a. "Oh, c'mon, honey, calm down."
   b. "I hate you, too!"
   c. "What exactly do you mean by that?"

2. **Your son wakes crying from a nightmare. Your first reaction is to**
   a. hug him tight and comfort him.
   b. tell him to shut up, big boys don't cry, and is he some kind of fruit or what?
   c. say, "Hmmmm. That crocodile nightmare again—a repetitive motif. Would you like to discuss what happened to you today in the sandbox?"

3. **A stunning woman in a revealing black evening dress enters a crowded cocktail party.**
   a. You watch her in fascination.
   b. You nudge your buddy and say, "Hey, I wouldn't kick that dame out of bed for eating crackers!"
   c. You watch the reaction of the men in the room as she enters, and the reaction of the women in the room to the men, and the woman's nonchalant reaction to the disturbance she has created. And then you say something pithy about the harnessed Id resulting in the great masterworks of Art and Music.

Key:
If you answered a to every question: You have no pretensions to deep insight into what people think, or why they do the nutsy things

they do. Skip psychiatry and find a nice, normal, healthy specialty that won't leave you questioning and endlessly evaluating your every thought, statement, and encounter.

If you answered b to every question: You have *no* sensitivity. Although this prevents you from being a decent human being, it does indicate your impeccable qualifications for being a Surgeon. Go back to Part One, or go cut up some dogs, because you've found your calling in life, and the person reading this to you doesn't have to keep reading aloud.

If you answered c to every question: Okay, okay, *be* a Psychiatrist! Even though it will kill your mother, who only wanted that you should be a Brain Surgeon, and who even now is slaving in the deli at home to put you through medical school. Go ahead! Hurt her! That's what you want to do, isn't it?

Pathology

There is a saying in medicine:

> Surgeons know nothing but do everything.
> Internists know everything but do nothing.
> Pathologists know everything, and do everything, but all too late.

You are a natural great pathologist if

1. you like the idea of saying, when the hospital calls you at home in the middle of the night: "Just put the patient in the freezer, I'll be there in the morning."
2. you prefer to deal with people when they are dead or cut up into small pieces.
3. you have established a meaningful relationship with your microscope.
4. you just *love* always having the last laugh.

Radiology

Along the lines of the popular bumper stickers TEACHERS DO IT WITH CLASS and NURSES DO IT WITH PATIENCE, there is a saying about radiologists:

> Surgeons do it.
> Internists talk about it.
> Radiologists just like to look at the pictures.

You should give Radiology serious consideration if you can honestly answer *yes* to these questions:

1. Do you like small, dark rooms in the basement?
2. Do you prefer to deal with pictures of people rather than the people themselves?
3. Do you feel terrific, not guilty, when leaving the hospital at 5:15 P.M. every day?
4. Are you unfazed by the prospect of glowing in the dark?

Pathology

"Oh, dear..."

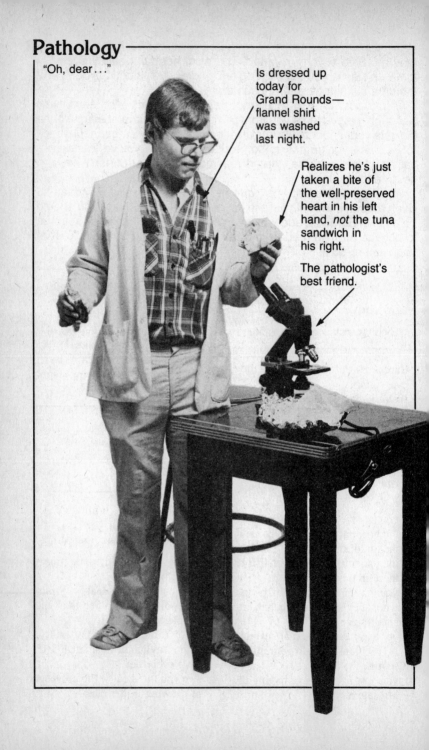

Is dressed up today for Grand Rounds—flannel shirt was washed last night.

Realizes he's just taken a bite of the well-preserved heart in his left hand, *not* the tuna sandwich in his right.

The pathologist's best friend.

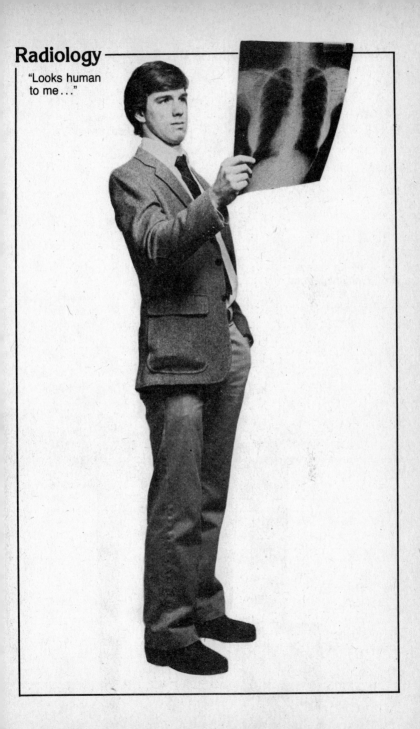

Radiology

"Looks human
to me…"

Dermatology and Its Wares

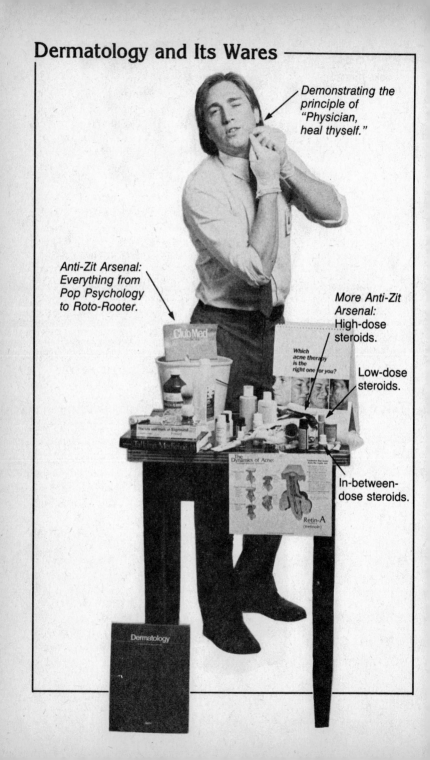

Demonstrating the principle of "Physician, heal thyself."

Anti-Zit Arsenal: Everything from Pop Psychology to Roto-Rooter.

More Anti-Zit Arsenal: High-dose steroids.

Low-dose steroids.

In-between-dose steroids.

Dermatology

Would you thrive in Dermatology?

1. Do you cope well with ridicule?
2. Can you refrain from punching out people who call you a pimple doctor, a superficialogist, or worse?
3. Can you get excited about acne craters?
4. Can you stay awake through articles on foot fungi?
5. Do you feel able to deal with neurotic women who are sure that their lives are being destroyed by submicroscopic skin imperfections?

If you can answer yes—sincerely—to these questions, Dermatology just may be the specialty for you, in which case you will need:

Principles of Dermatology

If it's wet, dry it.
If it's dry, wet it.
If neither of these works, use steroids.
If steroids don't work, do a biopsy.

Family Practice

Family practitioners are the workhorses of medicine—generally regarded as reliable, dedicated, hardworking, but none too bright.

Family Practice is for you only if you can answer *yes* to the following:

1. Do you like the idea of being a prominent upstanding member of a small town, serving on the local school board, and playing poker Thursday nights with your cronies—the town judge, the mayor, and the Deere tractor salesman?
2. Do you prefer a Cadillac to a Mercedes? Virginia Beach to Martinique? Golf to squash? Peas to asparagus? John Wayne to Dustin Hoffman? *The Guns of Navarone* to *La Cage aux Folles*?
3. Do you enjoy weekly visits from little old ladies who have no real ailments but count their visits to you as a significant social outing?
4. Do major traumas, very sick patients, big-time medical complications, and being home late for dinner give you acid indigestion?

A surgeon, an internist, and a family practitioner go duck-hunting.

The surgeon sees a duck, shouts, "Duck!" and shoots it down.

The internist sees a duck, shouts, "Duck! Rule out quail! Rule out pheasant!" and shoots it down.

The family practitioner sees a duck, and blasts it out of the sky with a round of machine-gun fire. As the tattered carcass falls to the ground, he remarks, "I don't know what the hell it was, but I sure got it!"

Family Practice

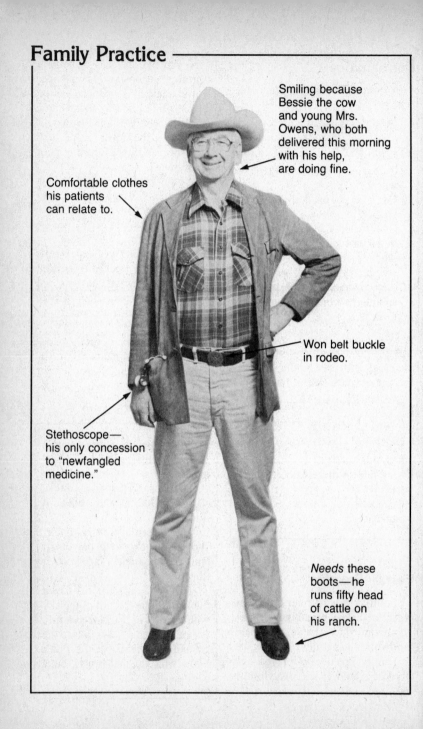

Smiling because Bessie the cow and young Mrs. Owens, who both delivered this morning with his help, are doing fine.

Comfortable clothes his patients can relate to.

Won belt buckle in rodeo.

Stethoscope— his only concession to "newfangled medicine."

Needs these boots—he runs fifty head of cattle on his ranch.

Ophthalmology

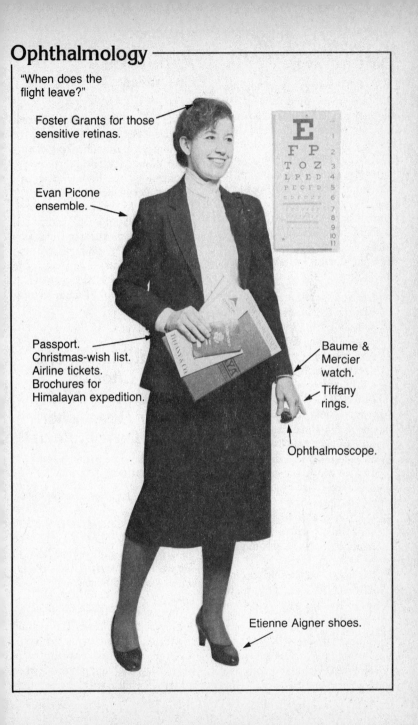

"When does the flight leave?"

Foster Grants for those sensitive retinas.

Evan Picone ensemble.

Passport.
Christmas-wish list.
Airline tickets.
Brochures for
Himalayan expedition.

Baume & Mercier watch.

Tiffany rings.

Ophthalmoscope.

Etienne Aigner shoes.

Ophthalmology

Ophthalmology is clean, neat, pleasant, diversified, and reasonably lucrative. Ophthalmologists, had they not gone into medicine, would have gone into international finance, the Foreign Service, or interior decorating. As a group, they are sophisticated, well-read, and masters of conspicuous consumption. Arthur Conan Doyle, Renee Richards, and Robin *(Coma, Fever, Brain)* Cook are but three of the more unusual doctors who chose Ophthalmology.

1. Do you love technically challenging fine work, such as exactly adjusting the second hand of your Baume & Mercier watch?
2. Are you capable of subtle distinctions, such as differentiating Château Lafite-Rothschild '57 from '59?
3. Do you love challenging diagnostic dilemmas, such as figuring out, while stranded on Grenoble's most difficult trail, exactly why you can't get the ski brake on your right Rossignol F-5 to retract?
4. Do you deal well with people, especially maître d's, chauffeurs, bellhops, and foreign ambassadors?
5. Do you want to help the medically underserved, especially those living on or near Central Park West?

If these questions elicited a rousing "certainly," you are without doubt prime Ophthalmology material.

All Those Other Specialties...

This is just the tip of the iceberg.

Medicine offers many pleasant subspecialties, like Ultrasound or Angiography, Bloodbanking or Surgical Pathology, Endocrinology, Neonatology, or Radiation Oncology, or Occupational Health.

You could do insurance physicals. Or be the doctor for the Chicago Bears. Or write a medical self-help column. Or volunteer to be the ship's doctor on *Love Boat*. The doors of medicine are open wide. Are you going to let them slam in your face?

Natural History of a Career Choice: Joe Gunner—NIH Cancer Researcher to Aspen Dermatologist

Childhood:

Joe goes to science, not tennis, camp.

Joe visits Washington, D.C., with his fourth-grade class, but when the class heads for the National Zoo to see the funny pandas, Joe splits for the Museum of Science and Medicine.

Instead of the Bruins or Red Sox, Joe has photos of Lewis Thomas and Sidney Farber hanging in his room.

Other children answer "fireman," "lawyer," or "postman" when asked what they will be when they

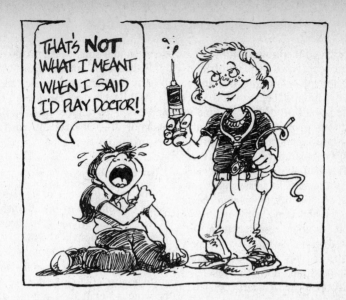

THAT'S **NOT** WHAT I MEANT WHEN I SAID I'D PLAY DOCTOR!

grow up. Joe answers, "Cancer researcher at Sloan-Kettering."

Joe's Science Fair project wows the judges (and he only used a little equipment from his dad's lab and got a little advice from his dad's graduate students).

Anxious about getting into medical school, Joe requests that his parents send him to Exeter so he will get into a good college for pre-med.

Adolescence:

Joe's nickname at Exeter is "The Doctor."

He makes varsity basketball, but prefers to bench-warm so he can pick up professional lingo from the team doctor.

He gets a job (with help from Dad) as an orderly at a local hospital for the summer, and steals a set of scrubs that he wears everywhere.

He never misses an episode of *M*A*S*H*, and eagerly deciphers Hawkeye's and B.J.'s back-chat about Kelly clamps, toothed forceps, and 4'0' catgut by watching with Sabiston's *Textbook of Surgery* on his lap.

He spends most of his time agonizing about college: Which college has the greatest number of premeds who go on to medical school? Which college has the greatest number of pre-meds going to the most *prestigious* medical schools?

College:

Rust never sleeps, and neither does Joe.

He becomes the most ferocious pre-med Stanford has ever seen. He takes Organic Chemistry in the summer school of a backwater college in Ohio to maximize his chances of an A +. He psychs out the competition in the toughest lab courses by arriving ten minutes early with a neatly typed summary of last night's reading and the protocol for the lab experiment (typed by his girlfriend, a Sociology major who is doing it "for the future, Joe").

He spends all of his free time in a famous professor's laboratory. After three years of steady labor, he finally comes up with some significant, publishable data. The very day that he Federal Expresses the summary of his work to *Immunochemistry,* he picks up a copy of *Science* and reads about researchers at Rutgers *(Rutgers!)* who did his experiment, in less time, with better equipment, and definitive results.

Scooped by Rutgers *(Rutgers!* Not even Harvard! What humiliation!), a disheartened Joe cancels his applications to graduate school and applies for medical school. So much for basic science research. So much for cancer. Someone else will have to figure it out.

Medical College:

Poor Joe Gunner has a tough time in medical school.

He's too smart for the surgeons. He conjugates his verbs, regularly uses polysyllabic words and subjunctive clauses, and asks too many questions they can't answer. He makes them very nervous. They are glad when he finishes the surgery rotation.

He's too unconventional for the internal medicine doctors. He refuses to pay lip service to the hierarchy. He points out to Attendings that their quotations from Osler are trite. He doesn't pretend to read the journals and says *publicly* that stu-

dents should stick to the textbooks!

Pediatrics is out: He doesn't like healthy children, let alone sick ones.

And Psychiatry? He doesn't like depressed psychotics, alcoholics, and polydrug abusers, at least not on a daily basis.

Internship:

Joe postpones choosing a specialty by doing a flexible internship.

Unfortunately, he goes through the same rotations and still doesn't like anything enough to do it every day for the next forty years. He feels just about ready to give it all up and become a detail man for the drug companies, or maybe do insurance physicals. . . .

But! On a ski vacation in Colorado he meets a bunch of dynamic, smart, friendly dermatologists who practice in the morning and schuss in the afternoon. They invite him out to do Dermatology and ski with them for a few months.

Joe has an excellent time with them. He decides to devote his life to battling the Heartbreak of Psoriasis . . . and to skiing.

Residency and Practice and Life:

Joe settles in Aspen with a thriving Dermatology practice and a charming ski-bunny wife, and lives happily ever after coping with zits, sunburn, and rashes. Every morning he faces a waiting room full of anxious, beautiful, adoring young women with microscopic skin imperfections. Every afternoon he hits the slopes!

CHAPTER 8

Specialists: An Inside Look

The Surgeon

Identifying feature: Enormous Ego.
Clothing:
  At Work
  • dresses in scrubs generally sprinkled with blood.
  • always wears comfortable sneakers with O.R. shoe covers.
  • white coat is generally grungy and unbuttoned.
  • wears mask down.
  At Home
  • never goes home.
Hobbies: Shoots ducks and stuffs them; trains hunting dogs; tracks caribou in Alaska.
Topics of conversation:
  1. His incredible feats of surgery.
  2. Surgical disasters (by *other* surgeons, of course).
Most frequent statement: (to O.R. nurse): "Dammit! Don't give me what I *ask* for—give me what I *need!*"

  He has *never* said, "I'm sorry," "I don't know," or "I was wrong." He has never actually *been* sorry. (He believes he's never been wrong.)

Most common worry: Something bad might happen to his fingers.
Favorite activity: Gossiping in the Doctors' Lounge between surgical cases.
Favorite magazine: Hustler.
Favorite TV show: The Dukes of Hazzard.
Last book read: Book? Has never *read* a book.
Most recent accomplishment: Recognized and treated a tension pneumothorax in the Emergency Room. To the astonishment of the slack-jawed medicine doctors, he slammed a Bic pen into the patient's chest, thus saving his life with prompt decompression (he has bored every crop of new Residents with a spirited retelling of this accomplishment).
Where does he shop? Abercrombie & Fitch, for his guns; wife buys all his clothes (he doesn't know where; he doesn't care).
Where does he eat? The Hospital Cafeteria 99 times out of 100, or steals food from the nurses' station and comatose patients' dinner trays.

  The other 1 in a 100 meals is eaten standing up, out of the refrigerator, when he gets home at

3 A.M. and the dinner his wife
saved has desiccated in the oven.
Where does he vacation? He
doesn't.

One Day in the Life of a General Surgeon: 6:15 A.M. to 9:53 P.M.

---

4 Hours: In the O.R., transplanting Mr. Sutton's brother's
kidney from Mr. Sutton's brother to Mr. Sutton.

3 Awful Minutes: Realizing that Mr. Sutton was supposed
to *donate* his kidney to his brother.

2 Hours: Building up courage to tell family.

4 Hours: In the O.R., transplanting Mr. Sutton's kidney
back to Mr. Sutton's brother.

30 Minutes: Yelling at Medical Students for being clumsy.

30 Minutes: Yelling at Residents for being clumsy.

45 Minutes: Yelling at O.R. nurses for being clumsy.

30 Minutes: Waiting for O.R. nurse to resterilize O.R.
equipment that surgeon has either dropped or
thrown at her.

20 Minutes: Rounds on 10 pre-op and 13 post-op patients.

1 Hour: Telling ribald jokes and gossiping with the nurses
in the surgeons' lounge in between cases.

1 Hour: Running down medicine doctors for being
spineless wimps.

1 Hour: Sleeping in Surgical Grand Rounds.

Grand Total: 15 hours, 38 minutes spent in the hospital—
just another routine day.

Surgeon

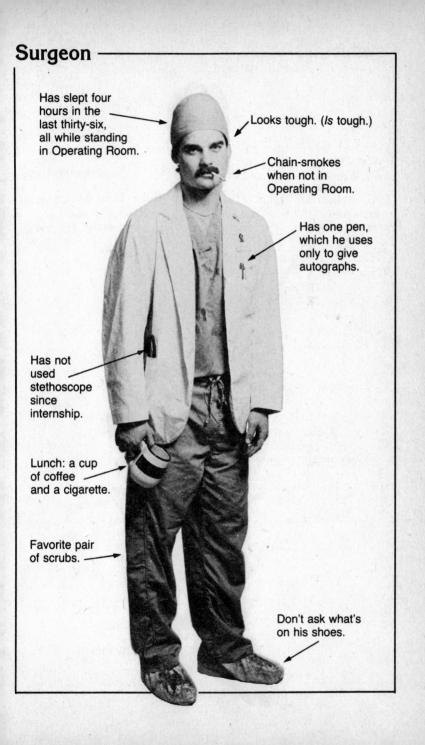

Has slept four hours in the last thirty-six, all while standing in Operating Room.

Looks tough. (*Is* tough.)

Chain-smokes when not in Operating Room.

Has one pen, which he uses only to give autographs.

Has not used stethoscope since internship.

Lunch: a cup of coffee and a cigarette.

Favorite pair of scrubs.

Don't ask what's on his shoes.

Psychiatrist

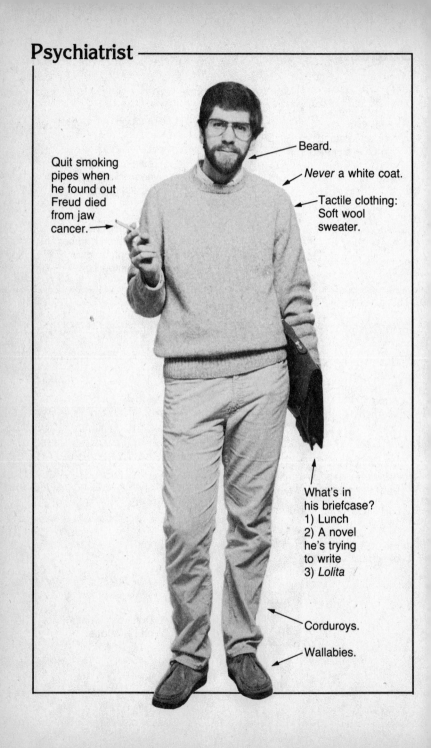

Beard.

Never a white coat.

Tactile clothing: Soft wool sweater.

Quit smoking pipes when he found out Freud died from jaw cancer.

What's in his briefcase?
1) Lunch
2) A novel he's trying to write
3) *Lolita*

Corduroys.

Wallabies.

The Psychiatrist

Identifying features: Ever-present low-tar cigarette; brooding silence or an unending flow of complicated sentences with many subjective clauses that are difficult to follow; conspicuous erudition.

Clothing:

At Work:

- comfortable, soft, natural fabrics.
- fisherman's cable knit cardigan or Shetland crewneck, never a white coat.
- overall effect is very paternal.

At Home
- Same as above.

Hobbies: Constant reading—of the highest quality. Writing—essays, novels, poetry. Contemplating—the universe. Speculating—what his relationship would have been with Freud.

Topics of conversation:

1. Therapeutic impasses.
2. How to cope with physically threatening patients.
3. How strange it is to be a marriage counselor going through a divorce (or an adolescent psychiatrist with a juvenile-delinquent son).

Most frequent statements:

1. "Hmm. And then what?"
2. "Can you tell me more about that?"
3. "Here's a Kleenex. It's okay to cry."

Most common worry: Who am *I* to say what's normal? Since when am I such an authority?

Favorite activity: Talking while someone *else* listens.

Last book read: Freud's *Interpretation of Dreams,* for the thirty-second time.

Most recent accomplishment: Gave a talk on psychoanalytic theory at the annual American Psychiatric Association meeting (in Vienna, of course!) that was *so* obscure only two other psychiatrists in the Western World could understand it.

Where does he shop? Spends most disposable income at local bookstore, to his wife's chagrin.

Where does he eat? Any Viennese restaurant will do.

Where does he vacation? He agonizes over the abandonment of his patients; he cannot bear to leave, but realizes that getting away is a must. Finally he compromises by telling everyone he's going away, but actually stays at home for two weeks (and gives his home phone number to particularly troubled patients).

The Pediatrician

Identifying features: Performing a physical examination on the floor; wrestling patient into mummy bag; has at least one stuffed toy on person at all times.

Clothing:
At work
- Brightly colored. Usually

One Day in the Life of a Psychiatrist: From 9:15 A.M. to 6:23 P.M.

1Hour: Cleaning, repacking, relighting pipe.
4 Hours: Encouraging patients to elaborate, including:

    537 uh-huh's
     82 "Can you tell me more about that?"
     77 "How did you feel about that?"
     32 restatements of fact as question
     28 encouraging gestures
     26 sympathetic nods
     11 "Lots of people worry about that."
      9 "No, I don't think those are crazy thoughts."

1 Hour: Dealing with angry patients, including:

      7 refusals to prescribe recreational psychotropic drugs
      5 denials of culpability for all that is wrong in patient's life
      3 reassurances that the therapy is indeed progressing even though the patient feels as anxious as ever
      1 rejection of physically seductive patient who then became physically threatening.

1 Hour: Dealing with angry family members, including:

      4 denials that psychiatrist told patient that all of his problems were due to his family
      3 reassurances that even though all of patient's problems are due to his family, it's not their fault
      3 explanations that even though all the patient's problems are due to his family, and it is their fault, there's nothing they can do about it now.

30 Minutes: Dealing with tearful, anxious people, including:

      1 long discussion with his wife about why psychiatrists have such rotten, screwy kids
      1 long discussion with rotten, screwy kid in question.

17 Minutes: Closing the 50-minute sessions

     19 "We're going to have to end soon."

14   "We'll have to discuss that in our next hour."

11   "We don't have time to get into that now."

50 Minutes: Talking with own analyst

31 Minutes: Serious self-doubts about ability to understand and treat diseases of the mind, about own state of mental health, and about whether Internal Medicine or Neurology might have been a better field to go into

---

Grand Total: 9 hours, 8 minutes, spent in office (does not include time at home ruminating about patients' problems).

The Pediatrician (Cont.)

stained. And always wash-and-wear.

- White coat with koala bears hanging on stethoscope, bright pins with holiday symbols (Easter bunnies, American flags, Halloween pumpkins)— all intended to divert the kids' attention from the instrument the Pediatrician is trying to use for examination.

At home

- Same, except for white coat.

Hobbies: Video games; Scout Leader; coaches the kids' swim team.

Topics of conversation:

1. Miss Piggy and Kermit the Frog jokes.
2. New video games on the market.
3. Creative Halloween costumes.
4. Diarrhea, asthma, otitis media, and failure to thrive.

Most frequent statement: "Mrs. Ei-

senmonger, just put the humidifier in her room, calm her down, and bring her around to my office in the morning."

Favorite activity: Selecting new toys for the office waiting room, and spending all afternoon "testing" the toys—for *safety,* of course.

Favorite magazines: Annals of Pediatrics, Ranger Rick's, Highlights.

Last book read: Golden Treasury of Baby Animals.

Most recent accomplishment: Successfully arranged federal funding for a night-time "well-baby clinic" to serve working parents, which has become extremely popular and heavily used.

Where does he shop? Toys "R" Us, F.A.O. Schwarz.

Where does he eat? Farrell's. McDonald's. Burger King.

Where does he vacation? Disney World. Seaworld. Disneyland. Sealand.

Pediatrician

Attempting a Physical Examination

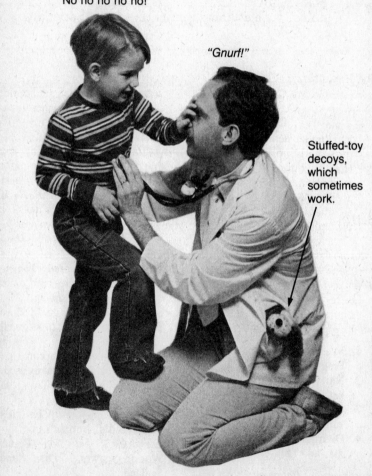

One Day in the Life of a Pediatrician:
9:15 A.M. to 7:00 P.M., plus phone calls all night long

3 Hours: Reassuring parents that the physical checkup is perfectly normal, and that their child is progressing exactly as he or she should be.

3 Hours: Trying to persuade uncooperative children to submit to a physical exam.

20 Minutes: Actually examining children

2 Hours: Telling kids that the vaccinations will hurt less if they don't move. Then telling them they moved.

10 Minutes: Grappling with a difficult diagnostic dilemma.

1 Hour: Discussing with nurse new ways to remove vomit stains.

15 Minutes: Sneaking out to the waiting room to covertly play with some of the neat new toys bought for the room.

Grand Total: 9 hours, 45 minutes (in the office).

The Academic Internist

Identifying features: Ramrod posture, tight sphincter control, tendency to lecture—everyone on everything.

Clothing:

At work
- immaculate, buttoned-up starched white coats.
- conservative rep ties.
- brown oxford shoes.
- pressed wool pants (even in summer in Atlanta).

At home
- pressed khaki trousers and Lacoste shirts, buttoned up.
- immaculately clean Pro-Keds.

Hobbies: Plays golf and tennis; keeps *exact* scores; knows all the scores from all his games in the last six years. Used to play ferocious squash, but his intensity made his squash partners so uncomfortable they quit playing.

Topics of conversation:
1. Internal Medicine.
2. Internal Medicine, Then and Now.
3. The Frontiers of Internal Medicine.
4. Why My Research Is on the Frontiers of Internal Medicine
5. Why Doesn't NIH Realize That My Research Is on the Frontiers of Internal Medicine?

Academic Internist

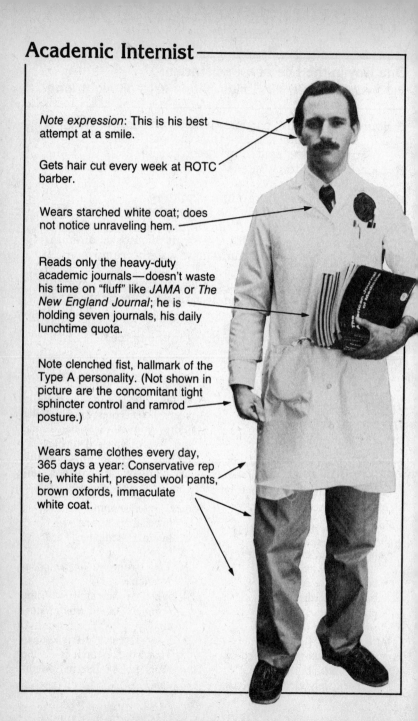

Note expression: This is his best attempt at a smile.

Gets hair cut every week at ROTC barber.

Wears starched white coat; does not notice unraveling hem.

Reads only the heavy-duty academic journals—doesn't waste his time on "fluff" like *JAMA* or *The New England Journal*; he is holding seven journals, his daily lunchtime quota.

Note clenched fist, hallmark of the Type A personality. (Not shown in picture are the concomitant tight sphincter control and ramrod posture.)

Wears same clothes every day, 365 days a year: Conservative rep tie, white shirt, pressed wool pants, brown oxfords, immaculate white coat.

Most frequent statement (to Residents): "Give us your Differential Diagnosis for this patient—and *skip* the ummm's and ahh's!"

Most common worry: His grant will dry up.

Favorite activities: Exposing the ignorance of Residents, discussing his research, tutoring his children in their math classes, "helping" his children with their Science Fair projects.

Favorite Magazines: Annals of Medicine, Science, Scientific American. At least four journals in his specialty, which he not only reads but also regularly contributes to.

Last book read: The Double Helix, in high school, which inspired him to go into research.

Most recent accomplishment: Was asked to write a review on his specialty for the *Annals of Medicine*.

Where does he shop? Brooks Brothers, or its local equivalent, for every item of clothing. He supervises his wife's selection of household items and has the final say on every furniture purchase. He does not require, but does prefer, that his wife document her food purchases and demonstrate that she selected the highest quality at the lowest price.

Where does he eat? At home, where he has full quality control over the food.

Where does he vacation? The Yucatán with his whole family; every day he schedules a two-hour family lecture session followed by individual presenta-tions by the children on Mayan civilization.

Greece, where the daily program calls for a three-hour lecture, two-hour individual presentation sessions, and then a three-hour forced march over the most obscure and challenging ruins.

He is quite surprised when his children indicate that they'd rather spend summer vacation with their doddering grandparents in Dayton, Ohio, than go to Italy on the next expedition.

The TV Soap Doctors

Identifying feature: Can always be found in the hospital cafeteria; never in their offices.

Clothing:

At work
- standard suit and tie for the men; revealing apparel for the ladies.
- over these stylish ensembles, a clean white coat devoid of cumbersome medical paraphernalia.

At home
- business suit; slinky silk lounging pajamas.

Hobbies: Golf, tennis, travels extensively. Never seen reading, holding, or owning a book.

Topics of conversation:
1. How's Alan taking the divorce?
2. Can Becca cope with alco-

One day in the Life of an Academic Internist: 8:15 A.M. to 8:45 P.M.

2 Hours: Reading the journals; writing for the journals; reading other Internists' submissions to the journals, rejecting them, smiling.

2 Hours: Directing hospital Rounds, demonstrating to the assembled medical students and residents just exactly how ignorant they are.

10 minutes: Teaching medicine in a nonpunitive fashion.

2 Hours: Ordering and interpreting tests for obscure and unlikely diseases.

1 Hour: Having lively arguments with other Internists over trivial details about these obscure and unlikely diseases.

1 Hour: Stomping off to the library to find and photocopy journal articles to prove his point about these diseases.

30 Minutes: Disparaging surgeons for being ignorant technicians.

30 Minutes: Complaining that surgeons make far too much, considering what they actually do.

30 Minutes: Regretting the decision to go into medicine and not surgery.

30 Minutes: Drafting an angry editorial for the *Journal of the AMA* on the inordinate amount of prestige and financial compensation awarded to surgeons.

2 Hours: Berating lab technicians in his research lab for being unproductive.

20 minutes: Actually having person-to-person contact with patients.

Grand Total: 12 hours, 30 minutes, spent in hospital, lab, and library.

The TV Soap Doctors (Cont.)

holism? Does Pam know of my passionate love for her?

3. Will Barb ever discover Bill's dark secret... and could she ever forgive him?

Most frequent statement: "Please ...we must talk about this, and X must never know that we know that he knows" (or some variation thereof).

Most common worry: See *Most frequent statement.*

Television Doctors:
Monica Quarterbrain, M.D.

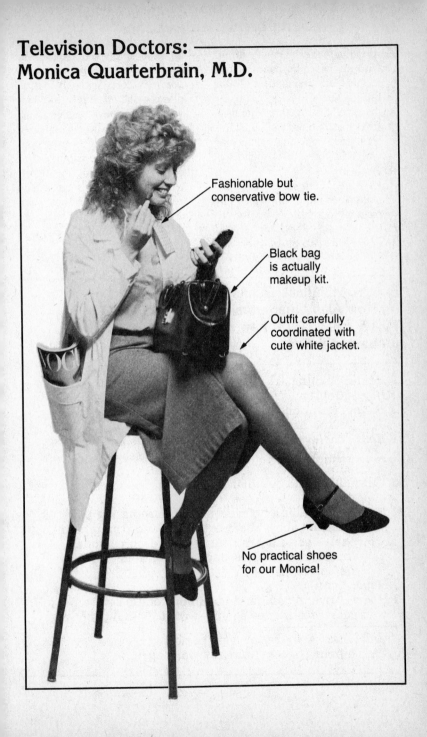

Fashionable but conservative bow tie.

Black bag is actually makeup kit.

Outfit carefully coordinated with cute white jacket.

No practical shoes for our Monica!

Favorite activities: Having affairs with the wives/husbands of colleagues, discussing these affairs, hiding these affairs, exposing these affairs, getting pregnant from these affairs and agonizing about abortion/adoption/keeping the child for several months of episodes.

Favorite magazines: Never seen reading, holding, or owning any medical journals.

Last book read: See *Hobbies.*

Most recent accomplishment: Had an affair and talked about .. it.

Where does s/he shop, eat, vacation? TV doctors go only to three places—the *hospital cafeteria,* where they have embarrassing encounters with their paramours; *home,* where they discuss their paramours and the paramours of others; and the No-Tell Motel, where they sow the seeds of evil gossip, among other things. They do not shop, eat out, or vacation.

How Your Patient Thinks You Spend Your Day; or, How Alan Quarterbrain Spends His Day: 10:15 A.M. to 2:00 P.M., with time off for protracted lunch

---

2 Hours: Fooling around with nurse at No-Tell Motel.

1 Hour: Golfing.

2 Hours: On phone with stockbroker, interior decorator, Billing Associates of Manhattan, Inc.

1 Hour: Involved in thrilling dramas of life-and-death illnesses with last-minute discoveries of cancer cure.

30 Minutes: Time out to accept Nobel prize for cancer cure.

1 Hour: Enthralling hour spent with fascinating patients, learning about the heartbreaks and triumphs in their lives, understanding their deep personal longings and hopes, and treating their hemorrhoids.

1 Hour: Tennis.

1 Hour: Drive to palatial home in one of his several Mercedes-Benzes equipped with TV and telephone.

Grand Total: 4 hours (or less) in hospital; 1 hour (or less) actually working

---

Television Doctors:
Alan Quarterbrain, M.D.
Need we say more?

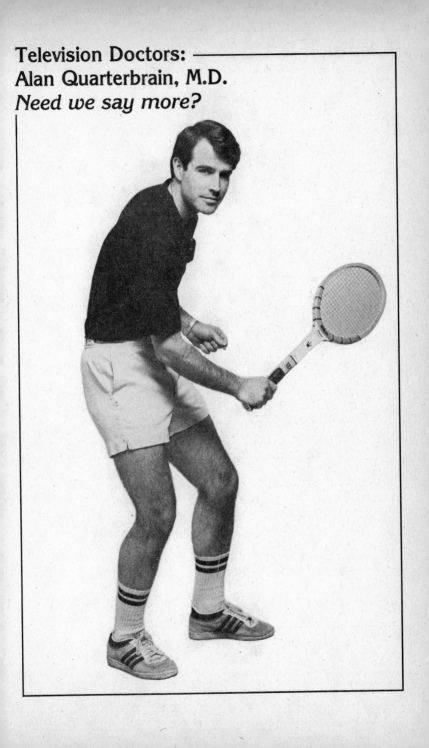

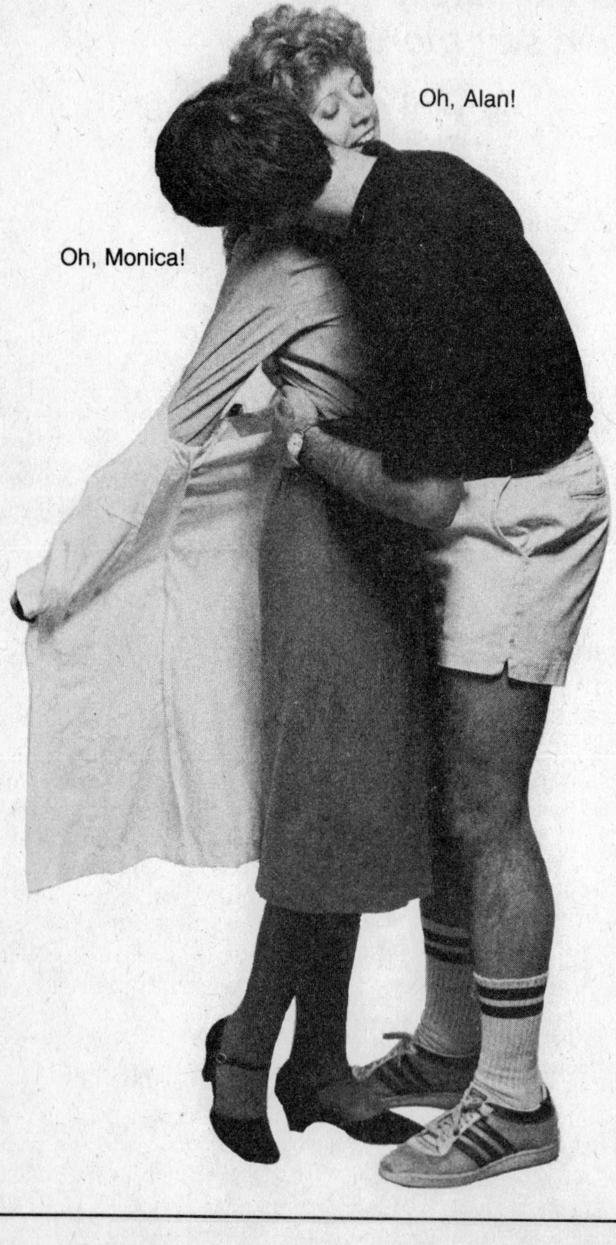
Oh, Alan!
Oh, Monica!

CHAPTER 9

Looking for a Residency in All the Wrong Places

The Hospital Recruiting Game

Go into it with both eyes wide open: The Massachusetts General, the Mayo Clinic, Stanford, and Parkland hospitals do not recruit Residents. *You* go to *them* on your knees, at which point they toss out your application unless you are a genuine preppie, Ivy Leaguer, Phi Beta Kappa, and your mother registered you at birth for the residency.

Who does recruit? Little-known hospitals, like St. Mary Immaculata Aseptica in Braunwald, Arkansas, or Joe's Bar and Grill and General Hospital in Moosehead, Vermont. Their need for Residents is desperate, so beware the exaggerations of their brochures:

• *"Great Recreational Opportunities":* means that the nearest library, movie theater, and shopping center are 60 + miles away, and you will be stranded in the deserted wilderness where the only forms of entertainment are snow-

mobiling, ice-skating, and trying to get more than one channel on TV.

• *"We maintain a close relationship with a major medical school"* means that they're both in the same city, and you can stop in and eat at their coffeeshop anytime you want.

• *"Very liberal benefits":* The top programs consider liberal benefits to be malpractice insurance, an on-call room, and all the white coats you can wear. Less prestigious programs might offer membership in the local golf club or two weeks of paid vacation. Really crummy programs will try to entice you with everything from bedroom furniture sets to an all-expense-paid trip to the Bahamas.

Be *very* suspicious of any program whose brochure:

• has *no* pictures of the hospital
• has a P.O. Box return address
• lists no American names on the hospital staff

99

Name That Hospital!

Hospitals frequently have nicknames intended to reflect the nature of the staff or the patient type.

Can You Match the Hospital with the Nickname?

Massachusetts General	Outer Limits
Beth Israel	The Slammer
Veteran's Administration	Massive Genitals
Good Samaritan	St. Elsewhere's
Our Lady of Mercy	The VA Spa
Our Lady of Holiness	Our Lady of the Highway
St. Elizabeth's	Beth Miserable
Outer Drive	Our Lady of Money

One day in Boston a man leaped into a taxi, grimacing in pain and clutching his groin, and shouted, "Take me to the hospital!"

"Peter Bent?" asked the cabbie.

"Bent?" the man yelled, "I think she bit it *off!*"

Fear and Loathing on the Interview Trail: A Crash Course in How to Interview for Residency

1. Clothing:
Always wear some.
Sumer's rule of thumb: Never dress better than the person who is interviewing you. Remember that surgeons have execrable taste in clothing and are themselves comfortable only in loose-fitting, blue-green, pajamalike outfits with drawstring trousers. A loud K-Mart tie and Sears finest polyester leisure suit, preferably with clashing checks and stripes, will get you noticed. But if you're interviewing for Radiology, call Ralph Lauren for an emergency consult, study *Gentlemen's Quarterly,* and prepare to buy a suit that will cost twice as much as your microscope.

2. Interview Etiquette: Waiting with the Other Candidates.
Growling at the other candidates is considered excessive.

Practicing the artful psych-out, however, is a delightful way to pass the time:

1. Tell the person on your right that no one from his medical school

Fear and Loathing on the Interview Trail: How to Dress for Your Radiology Interview

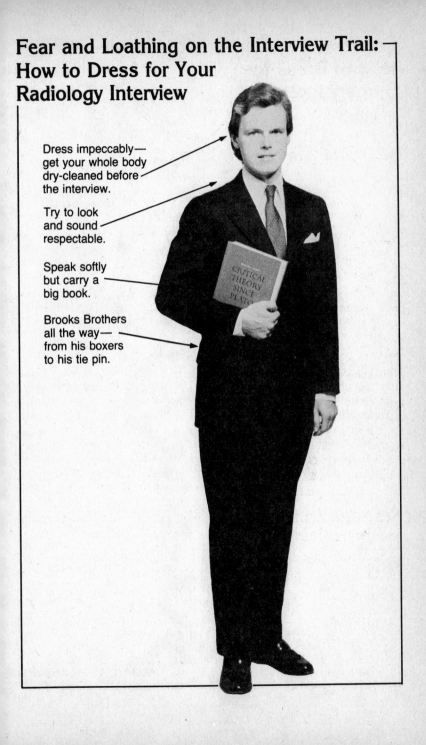

Dress impeccably—get your whole body dry-cleaned before the interview.

Try to look and sound respectable.

Speak softly but carry a big book.

Brooks Brothers all the way—from his boxers to his tie pin.

Fear and Loathing on the Interview Trail: How to Dress for Your Surgery Interview

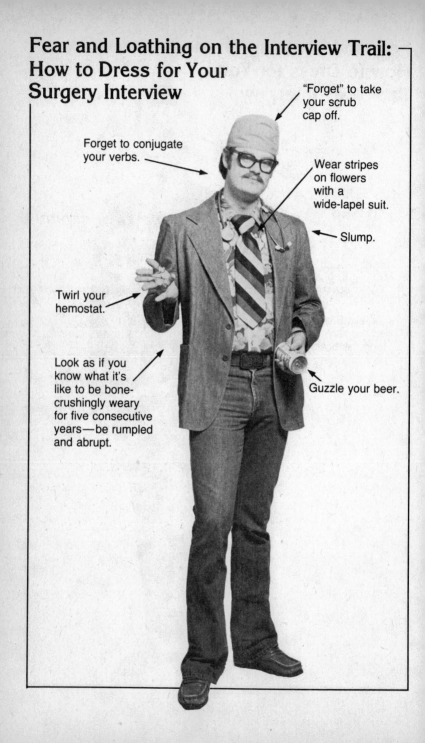

"Forget" to take your scrub cap off.

Forget to conjugate your verbs.

Wear stripes on flowers with a wide-lapel suit.

Slump.

Twirl your hemostat.

Look as if you know what it's like to be bone-crushingly weary for five consecutive years—be rumpled and abrupt.

Guzzle your beer.

has ever matched at this program.
2. Tell the person on your left that your father-in-law is Chairman of the Department.
3. Speak softly but carry a thick book—like *Ulysses* or *Neurologic Differential Diagnosis*. (Just don't let your copy of *Hustler* fall out from between the pages.)

3. Interview Etiquette: The Main Event.

After waiting three hours with fifteen people as calm as Thoroughbreds in a starting gate—here you are, closeted with some faculty bigwig who is flipping casually through your application, his mind on lunch.

- Encourage the interviewer to focus on your good points: *Don't* bring up Obstetrics/Gynecology if your evaluation from that rotation says, "Grossly incompetent—I wouldn't let this bozo deliver my *mail.*"
- Give the correct answer to: "Why do you want to specialize in this field?" Hint: The correct answer is *not* "Well, it's easy, and lucrative, with great hours, and I'm basically a lazy person who works as little as possible."
- Give the correct answer to: "Do you plan to practice in this area?" *Hint:* Answer: "No! No! No! Why would *anyone* want to practice in suburban Boston or Georgetown when they could practice in Deadhorse, Arkansas?" The better candidate you are, the greater threat you will be in six years when you

are fully trained and capable of staying in the area, draining off their good patients.

Five Questions to Avoid Asking the Resident Who Is Conducting a Tour Around His Hospital

- Would you drink Jonestown Kool-Aid instead of having to do your internship again?
- How come you look forty-five but you're only thirty-two?
- Did you ever have a sense of humor?
- Can you remember your kids' ages?
- Did you have that jackhammer stutter, nervous tic, and stooped posture before you started your residency?

You Can't Always Get What You Want; or, How to Control Yourself When You Match at Your 13th Choice

Match Day. The day when the results of a giant national algorithm are announced, placing more than 10,000 senior Medical Students in internships. It can be a day of triumph, for those who match at famous programs, attractive cities, or in competetive specialties; it can also be a day of crushing disappointment. Either way, it's a public event—everyone finds out in a big auditorium-style announcement—so here are some tips on how to behave when you discover that you can't always match where you want.

1. Tell everyone that you'd *rather* be in Akron than San Francisco. Mention the latest San Francisco joke: "What do granola bars and San Francisco have in common?"—"They're both full of fruits and nuts."

2. Say you didn't *really* want to go into Gastroenterology. Tell gastroenterolgist jokes: "What's the definition of a sigmoidoscope?"—"An eighteen-inch tube with an asshole at both ends."

3. Refrain from punching out the creep who matched at Massachusetts General and is ecstatically running around the auditorium hugging, kissing, and slobbering all over your classmates. He'll get his, soon enough.

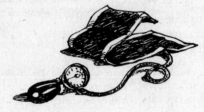

CHAPTER 10

The Intern's Survival Manual for Guerrilla Warfare

Internship: It's a Job, Not an Adventure

It's a dog-eat-Intern world out there.

No one has your interests in mind. The hospital will try to work you into the ground, the patients will insist on dying in the middle of the night (getting you out of a nice warm bed), and the staff, which is supposed to teach you, will instead ridicule you every day for your ignorance and sloth.

If you tried to do every chore they assigned to you in the *officially* proper way, you'd work twenty-five hours a day and *still* not finish your tasks as doctor, teacher, blood-drawer, administrator, orderly, and bootlicker. You'd probably wind up downing alternate fistfuls of Valium and speed, with a bleeding crater of a peptic ulcer and sleep-deprivation hallucinations.

So take some tips from guerrilla warfare, and protect yourself to ensure survival!

Make like wallpaper; or, *Why is the chameleon the mascot of the Na-* *tional Interns' Association?*—Visible targets attract work, that's why!

How to Admit a Patient—In Seven Easy Steps

Patients are like babies—they always arrive in the wee hours. You, of course, have to roll out of bed (if you ever got there) to find out what's wrong with them and start treating it, or "working them up." Your goal is to work them up as quickly and efficiently as possible and get back to bed, so you can cope with work the next day.

Step 1: When the phone rings in your call room, don't pick it up. Wait until the third, fourth, fifth ring—however many rings it takes to wake up the Medical Student sleeping in the bed next to yours. Then let him/her answer. The Medical Student's participation is critical in the success of this operation;

The Intern's Three Greatest Enemies

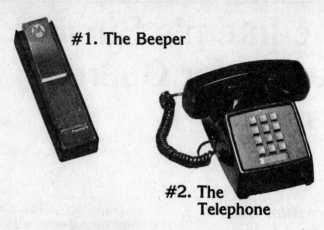

#1. The Beeper

#2. The Telephone

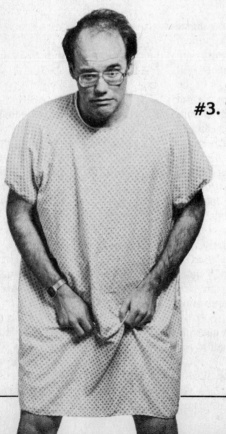

#3. The Patient

"Doc...I don't feel
so good...
did I tell you about
my constipation?"

some degree of consciousness on his/her part is therefore required.

If you cannot rouse your Medical Student, and you do have to answer the phone, identify yourself (if you can). One sleepy Resident answered the phone mumbling gibberish; when the floor nurse demanded, "Who *is* this, anyway?" she got the mumbled reply, "I don't know. It's too dark to read my name tag."

Step 2: Find the patient. This can be a trick in itself. At certain hospitals for old soldiers, patients have been known to disappear into elevators (or bars) for days.

Step 3: Remember the three critical questions every intern must ask his patient.

Number One: Are you a vet? If he is, turf him to the Veterans Administration Hospital STAT. If you do successfully send him off to the V.A., be sure to forward him under some other Intern's name, never your own. Otherwise, you will·win the eternal enmity of the Intern at the V.A. who receives your gift package in *his* hospital at 3 A.M.

Number Two: Which Intern took care of you last time? If Lady Luck smiles on you, the patient will be a "bounce-back"—i.e., some poor Resident spent all of May tuning up Mrs. Digoxin's congestive heart failure, but the day she goes home she eats a bag of potato chips and misses her pills, and boom—June 3 she "bounces back" to the hospital with ankles the size of tree trunks, unable to breathe, in fulminant congestive heart failure. The lucky

Resident's reward? He gets to take her back again. Your reward? You get to go back to bed, because you ferreted out the all important "bounce-back" connection. And don't bother to feel guilty as you trundle back to your call room, humming "Whistle While You Shirk." Your colleague will gleefully do the same to you at the first opportunity.

Number Three: Where is his chart from the last admission? This is where your semicomatose Student comes in handy—he/she can scout out the chart, which is chock-full of valuable information.

Worry when the Student says, "Do you want all thirteen volumes?"

Panic when the Student says, "I can find only six of the thirteen volumes."

Cry when the Student says, "I can't find *any* of the thirteen volumes," because then you'll be up all night, delving into long-forgotten history with a sleepy, sick patient.

Step 4: Read the chart. You wouldn't go to Paris without a Michelin guide. You wouldn't take the Los Angeles Freeway without a map. You wouldn't tackle an EKG without Dubin's. You wouldn't wander through the Himalayas without a Sherpa. Then why would you look at a patient without first studying his chart?

And be time-efficient. Send the Medical Student in to do a quick history and a thorough physical while you sit down, drink a cup of coffee, smoke a cigarette and attempt to decipher the chicken

Quiz: Will You Survive Your Internship?

Word Associations: cover the right-hand column of words; the closer your associations with the words on the left match those on the right, the better your chances for survival.

Patient . . . . enemy
Sleep . . . . unnecessary
Lab result . . . . not back yet
Student . . . . scutboy
Salary . . . . a joke

The most physically demanding work you've ever done:
   a. working on an Alabama chain gang
   b. Muhammad Ali's sparring partner in 1970–71
   c. longshoreman in Jamaica loading bananas from sunrise
      to sunset
   d. changing TV channels

Your tolerance for abuse, both verbal and physical, is
   a. outstanding
   b. incredible
   c. phenomenal
   d. nonexistent

Your goals for the coming year include
   a. staying alive
   b. avoiding severe depression
   c. not getting cut from the residency
   d. learning to play the piano, reading the newspaper every
      day, and taking up squash seriously

   Key:
   If you answered a, b, or c: You will probably survive internship with marriage, psyche, and career plans intact. *Probably.*
   If you answered d: You have as much chance of living through internship as your Gross Anatomy cadaver has of coming back to life as a whole person.

scratches your colleagues call handwriting.

Step 5: Now. Go look at the patient.

Verify any unusual findings the student has picked up.

Verify any findings the chart mentions—this will, by the way, impress your Student with your clinical acumen and thus foster troop morale, which generally flags in the small hours of the morning.

Step 6: Write it up.

Document that the fact-finding mission was indeed accomplished, and that there is *some* rationale for the treatment you embarked upon.

Send the Student off to draw blood, start an intravenous line, find the lab results, or look for X rays—this will save time, not to mention the opportunity to plagiarize shamelessly from the Student's write-up.

Chastise the Student if his write-up is not neatly written—only Interns and private practitioners scrawl.

Make sure that yours is illegible. Why have your mistakes and oversights in clear view for everyone to see?

Intern's note: L.O.L. in N.A.D. c/o T.B.F.; admit for Dx and Tx

Translation: Little Old Lady in No Apparent Distress complaining of Total Body Failure; admit to hospital for Diagnosis and Treatment.

Abbreviate like crazy. If there isn't an accepted abbreviation, make one up!

Step 7: Finally, write the admitting orders and hop back into bed.

Admitting orders cover every aspect of the patient's hospital stay: what room he'll go to, what he'll eat, special tests and treatments he'll require.

The first order generally instructs the staff where to send the patient, i.e., "Admit to Intensive Care Unit." In some grimier neighborhoods, however, the first order may be, "Bathe in the Emergency Room, *then* admit to 7West" or "douse in Kwell."

List the patient's medications. Remember, if you forget to list even the patient's daily Fred Flintstone vitamins, you may well get a midnight phone call from a harassed floor nurse with an irate patient who refuses to sleep until he gets his Freds.

List the patient's condition. Friends, relatives, and the media would all like to know if the patient is "good," "fair," "critical," or "pine box by bedside."

List the reasons why you would want the nurses to call you. Writing, "Call Resident if patient is dead" is a bit flippant.

Writing "Call Resident if you change your mind about Saturday night" is not exactly professional.

Writing "Call Resident after midnight if and when hell freezes over" is construed as uncooperative, and rude, to boot.

It helps if your orders make

sense—not always an easy feat on two hours' sleep when you're trying to keep the specifics of four newly admitted patients straight. Orders sometimes come out strangely. One sleepy Intern wrote:

ORDERS

1. ADMIT: to 7 East
2. CONDITION: good
3. DIAGNOSIS: unstable angina
4. DIET: regular
5. MEDICATIONS: bread
   eggs
   chicken
   milk
   call auto repair shop
   call bank
   call Mom

Once the orders are written—HEAD FOR BED! One patient admittal does not an immune Intern make; you must conserve your energy to cope with the inevitable rest of the night's disasters.

Other sections of the *Intern's Survival Guide,* available at any Survivalist Bookstore, include:

Troop Morale: Is every fourth Sunday off too much free time?

Heavy Artillery: Do you need a $150 stethoscope?

Jungle Health: Doughnuts as a food staple.

Fraternization with the ranks: Dating patients?

Fraternization with Residents: Diagnosis and treatment of trench mouth.

Residency: A Brief Description

Residency is just like internship except:

1. you are older.
2. you are more tired.
3. the thrill (such as it was) is gone, but the hours are the same.
4. Even your beeper fails to boost your adrenaline levels, now that you've learned to muffle it inside your jacket.

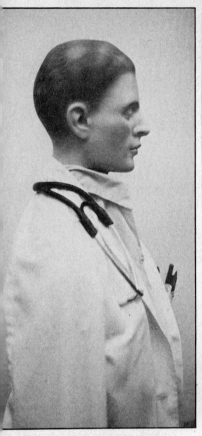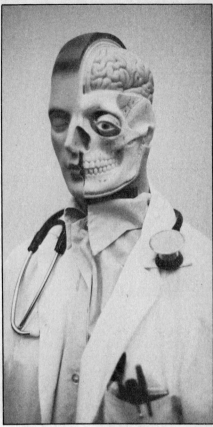

Intern, the night
before call

Intern, the night
after call

CHAPTER 11

Private Practice

You've endured medical school. Survived residency. Now comes the *hard* part—getting a job!

You have four options for practice: military, healthy-maintenance organization, solo practice, and group practice.

Military Practice

Did you really spend ten years in training so that some bureaucrat in gold braid who barely graduated from a military academy can order you around and transfer you at a whim to Thule Air Force Base in Greenland? Besides, military medicine requires extreme flexibility—try saluting while performing a rectal exam.

Health-maintenance Organizations

An ideal choice if you have a strong stomach for bureaucracy, like to call your patients "clients," and have an independent source of income.

Solo practice

There is one big problem with solo practice: finding patients. Patients will not, as you might have hoped; flock to your doorstep like shoppers at the start of Macy's Columbus Day Sale. You can't advertise, but you *can* make your presence more noticeable.

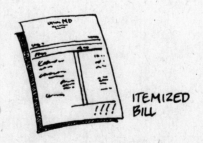

ITEMIZED BILL

General Announcement—The Madison Avenue Approach (on engraved ivory vellum)

Marcus Gunn, M.D.

with his freshly minted hotshot University credentials

wishes to announce

that he has arrived to work his modern medical miracles

for a select clientele

in

the practice of

OPHTHALMOLOGY

in the elite Palm Springs area

Consultation by *Appointment Only*	*22 The Atrium Offices* *Palm Springs*

The Bleeding-heart Liberal Approach to Professional Introduction   (on recycled paper)

Send Me Your Tired, Your Poor,

Your Huddled Masses Yearning to Be Treated Free.

Jacob Creutz Feldt, M.D. Equal Opportunity Medical Care

General Neurology

I Make House Calls

It's important to announce your presence to the general public and professional colleagues, but it is essential that you handle your introduction to your fellow specialists with kid—surgical?—gloves.

Specialized Announcements for Your Fellow Specialists (Xeroxed copy of typewritten announcement)

They will be none too pleased at the prospect of *more* competition; you must engage their sympathy by stressing your struggling practice.

Wilson Kimmelstiel, M.D.

A Poor Schnook with a Family to Feed and Debts You Wouldn't Believe

Just Wants You to Know

He's Setting Up a Practice Down the Street from You.

22 The Atrium Offices   Call & Talk
Sure, a fancy address but not so nice   I'm not busy
Palm Springs

If you are lucky, they will throw a few patients your way. Your newly employed secretary and file clerk might have something to do besides filing their nails.

Intra-office Politics: Thanking Quacks Who Refer Patients to You

Never steal patients. You can, however, diplomatically borrow them. Cover your tracks by sending your colleagues reassuring letters, stressing that you appreciate having patients referred to you and that you have not exposed their ludicrous treatments to the patient.

Ivan Rasputin, M.D.
Russian Imperial Court Plaza
& Shopping Mall
Las Cruces, New Mexico

Dear Dr. Svengali,

Thank you very much for referring this very interesting twenty-five-year-old white female to me, who obviously has been driving you crazy for the last four years with her multifaceted psychosomatic complaints, and who doubtless has never paid a doctor's bill in her life.

I treated her athlete's foot with a new antifungal agent, and I reassured her that the snake oil you'd been applying had probably not exacerbated the problem. I am enclosing an article you might do well to read, or perhaps you already have abandoned prescribing expensive placebos. The patient also mentioned to me that you performed an abortion for her in a most unusual fashion, which, if true, would greatly interest the State Medical Board.

Although I will foist this particular albatross off on the next sucker who attempts to set up practice in the area, I'd appreciate continued referral of any other patients you might spare.

Sincerely,

Ivan

Ivan Rasputin, M.D.

Group Practice

What is the most important thing to look for in choosing a partner? Age. Significant age.

Choose someone who is planning to retire or die soon, not some middle-aged M.D. who will meddle in your practice for the next thirty years. *Ask pointed questions:* How's his health? Does he get crushing chest pains when he lifts a reflex hammer, or does he run five miles every morning?

Why did the last partner leave? Was it an amicable parting? Or was it after a gunshot wound to the head over office receipts?

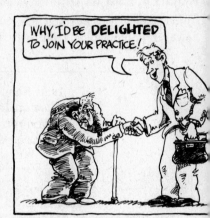

Avoid partners who...

...seem to have "mislaid" proof of their credentials.

...use the word "newfangled" in any context.

...start sentences with, "I may be old-fashioned, but..."

...have had more partners than the years they have practiced.

...come to blows with each other during your interview.

Don't join a practice where...

...the partners keep three malpractice lawyers on permanent retainer.

...payment is made in anything other than cash—chickens, cocaine, protection from the Mob.

...the waiting room has thick cobwebs.

...you're the only American-trained, English-speaking doctor they have been able to lure into an interview.

...there are bars on the windows and big signs on the door saying, "No drugs are kept in this office at night!"

Private Versus Public Practice

Private Practice is quite different from Public Practice, or Residency, as you can see from the orders written by Bob Lacrosse, M.D., as a Resident and later as a private practitioner in Obstetrics/Gynecology.

Public Practice: Internal Medicine

ORDER SHEET

10/10/69 2:15 A.M. (note time)
BATHE IN E.R.: with Kwell concentrate
ADMIT: to 5North/Internal Medicine

DIAGNOSIS: *the Dwindles (Nursing Home) says he hasn't been breathing much lately*

CONDITION: *one foot in grave/other on banana peel*

CHECK VITAL SIGNS: *don't bother.*

ACTIVITY: *not capable of any.*

DIET: *ensure liquid nutrient via nose-hose.*

MEDICATIONS: *Haldol*

LABORATORY STUDIES: *draw 2 quarts blood, send to lab in red-top tubes. Tomorrow morning we'll run every test the team can dream up.*

CALL HOUSE OFFICER IF: *patient dies.*

SPECIAL REQUESTS: *PBABS**

---

*Pine Box At Bedside.

Private Practice: Obstetrics/Gynecology

ORDER SHEET

10/10/82 4:15 P.M.
ADMIT: *to 5North/Gyn floor*

DIAGNOSIS: *Uterus in situ with Blue Cross/Blue Shield in purse*

OPERATION: *Elective hysterectomy in* A.M.

CONDITION: *Complaining*

CHECK VITAL SIGNS: Blood pressure q. 6 hours
　　　　　　　　　　Temperature, pulse q. 12 hours
　　　　　　　　　　Bank account q. 24 hours

ACTIVITY: Yammering on phone to friends about operation

DIET: The Scarsdale

DRESSINGS: Evan-Picone or Adolfo

DRAINS: only on my patience

MEDICATIONS: Valium, P.R.N. ad lib. (patient has own supply
　　　　　　　so don't even try to ration)

LABORATORY STUDIES: standard Blue Cross/Blue Shield Blue
　　　　　　　　　　Plate Workup

SPECIAL REQUESTS: she states that she will become emotion-
　　　　　　　　　ally incontinent if she does not get a pri-
　　　　　　　　　vate room with a color TV and good
　　　　　　　　　reception

CALL HOUSE OFFICER IF: 1. She complains of feeling ne-
　　　　　　　　　　　glected/anxious
　　　　　　　　　　　2. Her lawyer husband shows up
　　　　　　　　　　　and complains that she looks anx-
　　　　　　　　　　　ious and/or neglected
　　　　　　　　　　　3. She says *anything* like "I'm not
　　　　　　　　　　　sure I really need this surgery.
　　　　　　　　　　　Maybe I should postpone it, or get
　　　　　　　　　　　a second opinion..."

Thank you, Nurses!!

If M.D.s Could Advertise...

Lawyers do it shamelessly.

Hospitals and freestanding emergency centers do it.

Pharmaceutical companies have been doing it for years.

Rest assured, doctors are going to get into the act, soon enough.

Here's a sneak preview of what you'll see when doctors advertise:

The Mom-and-Apple Pie Politician's Approach

"My son is a good doctor and he wants to be your doctor.

Oh, sure, he's had all that fancy training at those big hospitals, and he keeps up with all the new technology. But the most important thing about my son is that he *cares*. He *cares* about his patients. Let him care about *you* and *your* loved ones. My son the doctor—Dr. David Wernicke-Korsakoff. The doctor who *cares*."

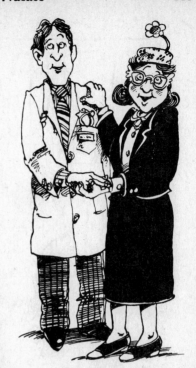

THE MOM-AND-APPLE PIE APPROACH

The Crazy Eddie Gotta-Sell-Those-Stereos Approach

"They call us crazy but we don't care!

We're surgeons and we love to cut!

We'd do it for free if we could!

We'll operate on anyone for any reason! Or for no reason at all!

DON'T MISS THESE SPECIAL SALES!

Gall bladders—50 percent off this week only!

Coronary Artery Bypass Grafts—HUGE DISCOUNTS!

Labor Day Sale on all cesarian sections!

Big Savings on used and damaged artificial hearts!

Remainder Sale on obsolete hip prostheses!

SATISFACTION GUARANTEED! WE'LL PUT PARTS BACK IF YOU'RE NOT HAPPY WITH THE RESULTS! ASK ABOUT OUR SPECIAL WEEKEND DISCOUNTS! CALL US! WE'LL TALK DEALS! ACT NOW! THIS OFFER WON'T BE REPEATED UNTIL NEXT WEEK!"

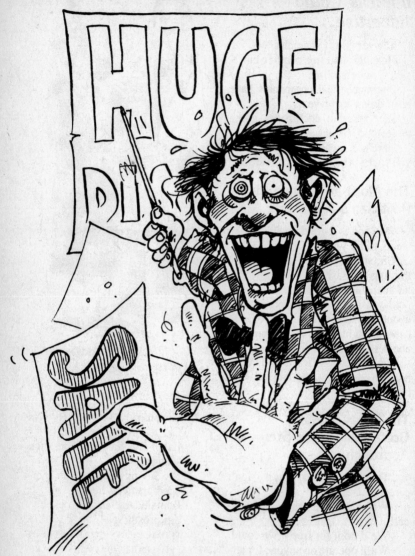

THE CRAZY EDDIE APPROACH

The Fast-Food Approach: Stressing Consistency, Economy, and Efficiency

♫ Take your leg off, take ♩
your heart out,
♩ Special procedures
don't upset us, ♫♫
All we ask is that you
♫♫ let us, ♪
Operate our way!

FIRST PATIENT: "The great thing about SurgiQuick is that you know exactly what you'll get, and how much it will cost, ahead of time."

SECOND PATIENT: "And it's so cheap! You get a full operation, and you still get change back!"

PERKY NURSE: "Next! May I help you?"

FIRST PATIENT: "One gall-bladder removal, please. Hold the complications."

PERKY NURSE: "Anything with that, sir? We're having a special on incidental appendectomies—*and* you get to keep the Mickey Mouse glass it comes in!"

FIRST PATIENT: "No, thanks."

PERKY NURSE: "Okay! That'll be $499.95, please! Thank you! Have a nice day, and thank you for shopping Surgiquick!" (She yells into microphone) "One gall bag, hold the complications! Next! May I help you?"

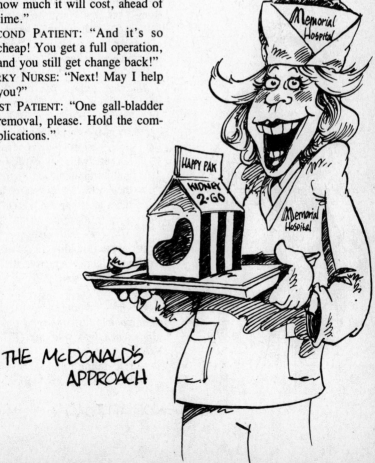

THE McDONALD'S APPROACH

The Snob Approach

"...Of course Cabot Surgical Associates is more costly.

Quality always is.

You don't skimp on the repairs on your Lear.

You refuse to compromise on the selection of your banker, your attorneys, even your tailor.

Why would you let someone you'd blackball at the club operate on your body?

At Cabot Surgical Associates, every surgeon is a squash-playing member of a good old-money family who prepped at schools you respect.

Cabot Surgical Associates—finally, surgeons for the truly wealthy...when you deserve the very best."

And What About the Drug and Medical-Supply Companies Advertising?

Pharmaceutical companies have already started advertising prescription drugs directly to consumers (with cents-off coupons and everything!) but that's just the tip of the iceberg. Watch for these commercial interruptions, coming soon on your own little screen.

Imagine an ad for prostheses along the lines of a designer jean ad.

(A gorgeous couple on horseback gallop along a beach at sunset, with an extra horse galloping alongside them. As they draw closer, you see large tubes attaching the horses, and a large machine on the back of the second horse.)

VOICEOVER (breathless): "Jodacke Artificial Hearts...to live the life you've only dreamed of!

Or how about surgical-equipment companies? Imagine this ad sandwiched into your Six O'Clock News.

(Operating-room scene—two harried surgeons working in-

THE SNOB APPROACH

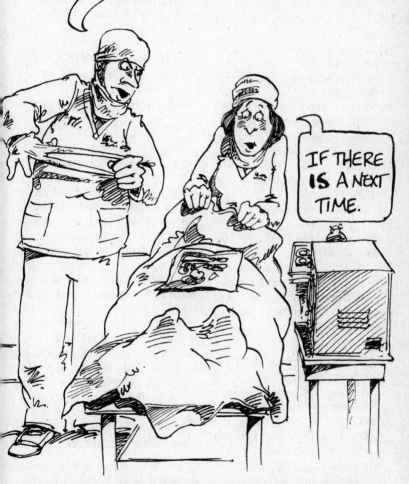

WHAT TO EXPECT WHEN PHARMACEUTICAL AND MEDICAL SUPPLY COMPANIES ADVERTISE

credibly hard; very tense music is playing in background, with a counterpoint of erratic heart-monitor beeps that are spaced farther and farther apart.)

ANESTHESIOLOGIST: "We're losing him! We're losing him!"

FIRST SURGEON: "He's still bleeding!"

SECOND SURGEON: "These sutures just won't hold!"

ANESTHESIOLOGIST: "He's gone! He's gone!"

FIRST SURGEON: "Dammit! We should have used Decathalon® sutures!" (He snaps off his gloves angrily and throws them down)

(Music and monitor abruptly stop: complete silence.)

VOICEOVER: *"Decathalon®* suture. Ask for it *by name."*

This ad would be ideal during the daytime soaps.

(Sobbing woman in the Intensive Care Unit waiting room; violins swell in background as stunningly handsome surgeon enters and puts his hand on her shoulder.)

SURGEON: "We did all we could. No one can be blamed. No one could have predicted your husband's ventilator would malfunction."

WIDOW: "But he was so young! So good! Our lives were barely started together. And my children—what can I tell them? How could the machine just not work?" (Violins swell.)

SURGEON: "I'll do all I can to help you through your troubled times."

(He looks deeply into her eyes as the violins saw away.)

"Has anyone ever told you . . . just how beautiful your eyes are?"

VOICEOVER: "This never would have happened if her husband had been attached to an Everworking Ventilator . . . Everworking Ventilators— aren't your loved ones *worth* it?"

Saturday Morning at Home with an M.D.

Scenario Number One: The Optimal Situation

Dr. Nieman Pick wakes up at 6:15, does twenty minutes of Royal Canadian Air Force calisthenics, drives to the hospital, where he rounds on his patients (only two today, thank goodness!, who are both doing well), discusses them briefly with the sleepy but pleasant Resident, writes a note indicating that his therapy is working, and gets home by 8 A.M., a full day of leisure ahead of him!

On this particular morning, his teenage daughter is riding in a local horse show, so he and his wife go to watch. She wins her first blue ribbon! A very full and satisfying morning all in all.

Scenario Number Two: The Usual Scenario

Dr. Nieman Pick rouses himself from bed at 7:15, refraining from pressing the snooze bar a third time. He drags himself over to the hospital to deal with three extremely sick patients, who kept him up until midnight last night and just haven't been responding to therapy. At fifty-five, he's just feeling too old for this! He gets to the hospital at eight, checks in on his patients, who are all doing terribly, discusses the cases with the equally baffled Chief Resident, and calls in a few specialists. The three specialists ponder the cases for a few hours, come up with some plausible ideas, and suggest some therapeutic measures, which work.

The morning is shot. Dr. Pick doesn't get home until 2 P.M., missing his daughter's horse show, where she won her first blue ribbon, but at least his patients are doing well and he'll be able to sleep tonight.

Scenario Number Three: Oh, God, Not Again!

Dr. Pick wakes up at 5:15 A.M. in the nurses' station of the Surgical Intensive Unit, where he fell asleep at 4 A.M. A nurse is gently tapping his shoulder, "Dr. Pick, I hate to wake you. Your patient is hemorrhaging again and the Resident needs to know if you'll take him back to the Operating Room." Dr. Pick groggily gets reoriented...he was in the Operating Room with this patient until midnight, trying to stop the bleeding from esophageal varices. "Yes, he's a young man, we'll take him back."

He and a team of Residents struggle to save the patient until 4 P.M., then give up. At 6, the patient stops breathing. Dr. Pick wants to cry, but instead falls asleep in the surgeons' lounge. His wife comes to get him

at 11, and he goes home to watch the Saturday Night Late Movie and drink a beer with her. At 6 A.M. on Sunday morning, he's back in the hospital, rounding on his remaining patients.

Why Do All Doctors in the Area Belong to the Same Country Club?

- They don't have to put up with snide comments during their Thursday-afternoon golf.
- Having the old beeper go off during dinner doesn't cause a ruckus.
- If they have to leave the Saturday Night Poolside Dinner Dance to go to the hospital, they can usually get a ride to the hospital from someone else who has also been called away. And their wives can drive home together if they don't get back.
- The chances of picking up a few referrals are greater if you play tennis with an endocrinologist, a pediatrician, and a surgeon every week, than if you play with two stockbrokers and a tax lawyer.

The Dr. and Mrs. Give a Dinner Party

Guest list: They are careful to invite noncompeting specialists—the last time they invited two general surgeons, all they did was glare at each other all night. And those two psychiatrists launched into a loud philosophical argument no one else even understood!

They'd like to invite someone outside medicine, but they only know one couple who aren't doctors—the broker and the advertiser who live next door—and it's getting a bit tiresome inviting them *every* Friday night.

Date and time: They have to be careful to tailor the time to the specialties—the last time they had an eight-o'clock dinner, the general surgeon they invited fell asleep on the couch over dessert. His wife was nonchalant—"Oh, Ken does this everywhere. Do you have a blanket? I'll cover him up and we'll go back to dessert"—but the other guests were flabbergasted.

Degree of formality: Always a sticky wicket. If they break out the Georg Jensen, will their guests think they're showing off? If they serve casserole will everyone think his practice is in trouble? Will everyone come in the wrong clothes, like that time when the radiologist came in a white Calvin Klein suit and the psychiatrist came in directly from restructuring his compost heap in his oldest and most pungent clothes?

The best dinner party they ever had: The night they invited five couples over to the local winery, where they "educated their palates" with a two-case wine-tasting marathon. At 2 A.M., the little old vintner, alarmed by their advanced state of inebriation, took it upon himself to drive everyone home, lecturing them on how they should be ashamed to be so smashed: "I can't believe

doctors would cavort and sing in the streets—it's *disgraceful!"*

The worst dinner party they ever had: When the Dr. invited his doddering partner and wife over for dinner—but forgot to tell the Mrs. So, at 6 P.M., she was halfway through her videotape "Workout with Jane Fonda," minus the leotard (because, hell, no one was at home), when the doorbell rang, and she called out, "The door's open, honey!" But it wasn't honey at the door.

They were able to laugh about it later—about two years and three Elsa Peretti necklaces later. His doddering partner's heart condition wasn't, unfortunately, aggravated by the surprise.

Dr. He and Dr. She (Try to) Give a Dinner Party

- They decide to entertain only because of the year's accrued social debts. They are *not* looking forward to this.
- They take a look around the apartment (which resembles war-torn Beirut, *not* a haven for gracious dining) and decide to have people over to a restaurant.
- They make reservations at a local restaurant and start calling friends—only six out of eighteen are free.
- The Big Night arrives, but she's hung up in the Operating Room with a ruptured aortic aneurysm and he's struggling to keep a preemie alive in the Neonatal Intensive Care Unit. He *does* take time

to call the restaurant, though, and the maître d' reports that their six friends are having an excellent time carousing without them.

- Neither of the doctors makes it to "their" dinner party, but later their friends tell them it was the best dinner they've been to in a long time.
- They are pretty sure there's a lesson there, somewhere.

How to Identify Doctors' Kids: The Hallmarks of an M.D., Jr.

- They charge when they play doctor.
- They're the only kids in kindergarten who raise their hands and say, "I gotta void."
- One zit and they've got biweekly appointments at the dermatologist.
- Doctors' kids are the first ones on the block to have:
  1. Glasses
  2. Braces
  3. Nose jobs
  4. IUDs
  5. Access to Valium
  6. Career plans (usually definite by kindergarten)
- In junior high, doctors' kids are studying for the SATs. In high school, they're prepping for the MCATs with Stan Kaplan. By college, they are branching out to one of four things:
  1. Developing anorexia nervosa.
  2. Terrifying nine-tenths of the pre-med population and collabo-

rating with the most brilliant one-tenth.
  3. Leaving for India on an adventure in self-actualization and creative drug abuse.
  4. Abandoning all career plans and taking dead-end education courses, but aggressively pursuing the most eligible pre-med on campus.

The Doctor's Kid Gets Married: Consolidation of Daddy's Referral Base

- It all starts by calling the Sunday *New York Times*. If the young couple doesn't get in, Dad calls the wedding off. Who wants such a socially insignificant person to join the family?
- The invitation list is *huge*, generally 500-plus. This is called "consolidation of the referral base"; the reasoning is that the next time a referral comes up, the specialist will think, "Oh, I'd better send this patient to Harry. After all, he *did* invite me to his daughter's wedding."
- The reception will be enormous, with lavish food and a thirty-piece big band, at the country club. It's important to demonstrate to the world that Daddy's practice is flourishing. No one wants to refer their patients to a failure, after all.
- The young couple is immediately catapulted to the upper-middle class, even if they were living before the wedding with brick-and-plyboard bookcases in a fifth-floor

How to Identify Doctors' Kids; First Ones on the Block with:

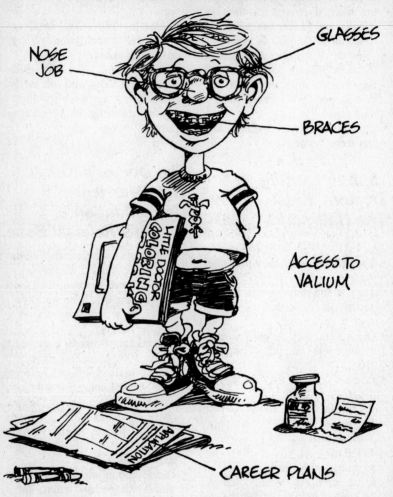

NOSE JOB

GLASSES

BRACES

ACCESS TO VALIUM

CAREER PLANS

walk-up. That's because Daddy refers patients, too, so the gifts that specialists give are substantial. The kids might still live in the fifth-floor walk-up, but they'll eat off Lenox china and Waterford crystal with dinner cooked in one of the six microwaves they got.

The Doctor's Mother Comes to Visit

She is disappointed when her daughter-in-law doesn't come to meet her at the airport, too. When the Doctor explains, "Mom, she has *her* practice, too; she's busy," Mom narrows her eyes and says ominously, "Too busy for me, eh? I don't have to be Freud to understand what *that* means."

When he explains that his wife will be on call that night, so they won't see her until tomorrow, she says, "Son, is your marriage in that much trouble?"

She is surprised by his old, beat-up car when they get to the parking lot. "What? You've been in practice for years and you're driving *that*?" When he explains that he really isn't making that much, and besides, day care, house payments, and his medical schools debts are not insignificant, she says, "Son, you can tell your mother. Your practice is in trouble, isn't it?"

She shakes her head when she sees his office. "Dear, don't you think your nurses should look more official? Wearing *uniforms* would be much better, with little hats." She is unfazed when he points out that the "nurse not in uniform" is actually one of his partners.

She boasts to his partners how brilliant her son was when he was in junior high, and how she always planned great things for him. *"Great things,"* she sniffs as she looks around the cramped waiting room of the unfashionable office, *"not this . . ."*

She shakes her finger at the surprised patients in the waiting room and admonishes them, "You better pay your bills—my son's kids are starving and he drives a foreign compact!"

She is amazed at dinner when his kids aren't unmannered Indians, and actually ask for the salt and pepper. "Well, I suppose the strangers who take care of them all day have taught them *something*." When the little ones actually go upstairs at the stroke of eight without prompting to brush their teeth, put on their pajamas, and put themselves to bed without help, she sighs, "Well, the poor children *have* to take care of themselves; they're practically *orphans*, after all."

She lectures her teenage grandson when she hears he's having trouble with high-school geometry. "You'll never get into Princeton with a D in math!" She gets chest pain when her Son the Doctor says maybe his son isn't Princeton material. She thinks she's having a heart attack when her grandson says, "Really, Grandma, Dad and I have talked about it. Maybe I'm just not college-bound at all. Maybe I'll sell organic vegetables, like Grandpa used to." She looks to the heavens and despairs. "For this we slaved so hard at the fruit market?"

When she returns to Miami, she boasts to her friends about her brilliant Son the Surgeon, his lovely wife—*also* a doctor, don't you know—and their well-behaved children, who cried to see Grandmomma go. "Here, let me show you the pictures—this one's Bill, he's in high school now, but we think he'll go to Princeton. . . . Oh, yes, he wants to be a doctor, just like his dad. My Son."

CHAPTER 12

Patients: A Field Guide to Wild Species

A WORD OF CAUTION

Approach these Big Game cautiously. Do not startle them. Under the slightest provocation, they, like the shortsighted rhinoceros, may charge or sue.

Anyone can be your patient. There are no restrictions, no qualifications, no screening exams. Look around the average New York subway car: two filthy drunks who might well be dead, three actively hallucinating little old bag ladies, two extremely dangerous-looking zonked-out punk rockers feeling the need for drug supplements, and a slew of fat, pale, overheated, none-too-clean-looking average Joes. Any one — or all, on a good day — can stumble into your nice neat office demanding that their needs be met. And they might not even be sick! Standing between you and that 450 SEL is a spectrum of problems ranging from tummyaches to imaginary tumors to leukemia. Your mission,

should you choose to accept it, is to ascertain the following:

1. What is their problem?
2. Can you fix it?
3. Can they pay?

(Not necessarily in that order.)

You may easily get stuck on Question #1. If you've ever been lost in Queens, or in the backwoods of Tennessee, or O'Hare Airport, you know how difficult it is to extract clear communication from the average man-in-the-street, who is often incapable of conjugating verbs in his native tongue, and whose conversation style consists of Sylvester Stallone-like multitonal grunts.

Getting a Medical History

A typical conversation:

DOCTOR: "What brings you here today?"
PATIENT: "I don't feel well."
DOCTOR: "Anything specific?"
PATIENT: "I feel rotten — terrible."

DOCTOR: "How long has this been going on?"

PATIENT: "Weeks, months—long time."

DOCTOR: "What made you decide to come here *today*?"

PATIENT: "I told you, I don't feel well."

DOCTOR (popping a Valium): "What exactly is the problem?"

PATIENT (irritated): "What, I got to do your work *for* you? *You're* the doctor, *you* figure it out!"

Review of Systems; or, Supplying Ammunition to Hypochondriacs

The hallmark of the suggestible patient is someone who has no focused complaint, but has a "completely positive" review of systems, as in this example:

DOCTOR: "Okay, now we're going to run through some general questions. Had any visual changes, like blurriness or poor eyesight?"

PATIENT: "Oh, yes, sometimes I can barely focus, it's awful... although right now I see okay."

DOCTOR: "Any changes in your hearing, ringing in your ears?"

PATIENT: "Sometimes I can barely hear anything, my ears get all clogged up. Maybe it's a brain tumor?"

DOCTOR: "Any dizziness, faintness, seizures?"

PATIENT: "Oh, I feel dizzy and weak all the time, I can barely move—not right now, though.

The acid test of the suggestible patient is an affirmative answer to either of these questions:

Does your urine glow in the dark?
Do your teeth itch?

Patients with itching teeth and glowing urine should be only briefly questioned before moving on to more concrete information gathering, such

---

Warning Signs That It's Going to Be a Long Interview

DOCTOR: "What brings you to the office today?"

PATIENT:

1. "Well, I wasn't very pretty as a child..."

2. "Why? Don't you *want* me here?"

3. "My car! Ha ha ha! Get it, Doc? My *car* brought me here!"

4. "Oh, it's a long story; it all started back at Aunt Polly's birthday party, back in '67 or '68—or was it at my mother's? Anyway, we were at this party— Come to think of it, it could have been a Christmas party, and not a birthday party at all. Anyway, my husband and I had just had an enormous fight, really knockdown, drag-out, and Harry, my husband— Well, he's not my husband now, we're divorced, and he's dead now— Doctor, are you listening?

as the physical examination and laboratory tests.

Understanding Your Patients: What Your Patients Say and What They Really Mean

What They Say	What They Mean
I'm worried about this mole.	Is it cancer?
I'm worried about this headache.	Is it cancer?
I'm worried about this lump.	Is it cancer?
I know this sounds silly, but...	Is it cancer?

The Doctor as Last Confessor; or, Why Patients Tell Doctors the Truth

The whole truth and nothing but.... This can be quite an eye-opener to those of us who attended single-sex Catholic institutions and married our high-school boyfriends.

For instance, the guy with the unusual venereal disease* is *not* going to concoct a story about unusual encounters with a toilet seat. No, sir. *You're* going to get the low-down about Plato's Retreat, in all its grimy glory. The facts may be shocking, but never lose sight of the fact that you are a *professional*.

- *Avoid judgmental statements* such as, "You *did* what? To *whom*? *How*? That's *bizarre*!" Yours is not to reason why, yours is just to diagnose and treat.
- *Avoid comments that reveal your personal naïveté* such as, "Wow! I didn't know that was anatomically possible!" Or "And what role does the German shepherd play?" Just get the facts.

Remember, the patient has everything to gain and nothing to lose by telling the truth. *You're* not going to punish him with twenty Hail Marys, or threaten him with divorce, or tell him he's going to get hairy palms. *You're* going to give him some bi-buttock intramuscular penicillin and send him on his way!

Lay Variations on Medical Terms

What They Say	What It Was
Fireballs in my eucharist	Fibroids in my uterus
Sick-as-hell anemia	Sickle-cell anemia
Smiling Mighty Jesus	Spinal Meningitis
Very close veins	Varicose veins
Flea bites	Phlebitis
Pabst test	Pap test
B-9 tumors	Benign tumors
High blood	Hypertension
Low Blood	Anemia
Cadillacs	Cataracts

*Venereal Diseases are now called Sexually Transmitted Diseases, or S.T.D., which frequently confuses people who don't understand how they got motor oil from a one-night stand.

CHAPTER 13

Those Strangers to Whom You've Dedicated Your Life: Your Patients

Patients fall into a few main categories. Most types are benign but irritating, like the common cold; a few are grossly malignant and best avoided at any cost.

The Chronic Complainer; or, 101 Vague Complaints

These people don't have medical histories, they have *sagas*. Classically the Chronic Complainer is a well-to-do suburban lady who has "Generalized Dissatisfaction with Her Life"—too little to do and too much time to do it in. Mrs. Munchausen will complain of headaches, weakness, dizziness, diffuse abdominal pain, backaches, and other nonspecific, nonreproducible complaints.

You can diagnose it, but you can offer her no cure.

She will leave your office angry and disappointed, but don't worry. She'll be back.

The Professional Patient; or, Recreational Medical Illness

The definitive sign of the Professional Patient is anyone who comes into your office looking healthy as a Budweiser Clydesdale but carries a chart more than one inch thick.

Other characteristics of the Professional Patient:

1. She has seen more than four doctors in the last year for the same medical problem.
2. She chats with great enthusiasm about horrible symptoms (vomiting, bloody stool, excruciating abdominal pain), but looks healthier than you do.
3. She says one of the following:

   • "My last doctor just didn't understand me." (Chances are good that you won't either.)
   • "I was unhappy at the Mayo Clinic." (Mostly because they

The Chronic Complainer

Oh, my head!

Oh, my back!

Oh, my feet!

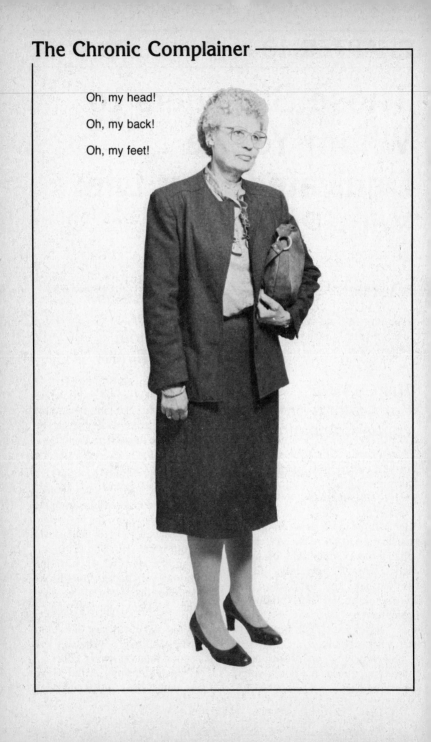

The Professional Patient

Looks healthy as a Budweiser Clydesdale...

But is carrying an eight-volume medical record into your office... complete with serial EKGs from 1947

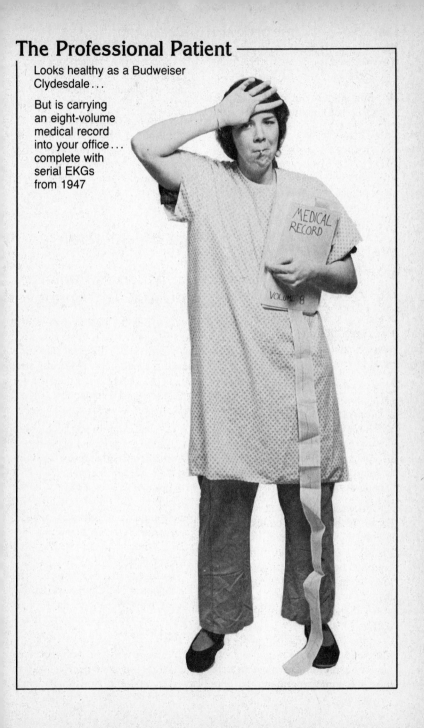

refused to give her an exciting and dramatic diagnosis.)

4. She stomps out of your office when you mention these words:

- further testing is really unnecessary
- your previous workup was excellent
- perhaps psychosomatic illness
- I can refer you to an excellent psychiatrist

The Medical Expert; or, Self-diagnosis by the Average Joe

This guy will stumble into your Emergency Room, announce his diagnosis, and demand a specific surgical procedure:

- "Doc, my stomach is killing me. I've got appendicitis. You've got to operate, now!"
- "I have a terrible headache, I need a CT scan!"
- "Give me some penicillin. I've been coughing all week; I've got pneumonia."

The problem with the Medical Expert is that he will be resistant to any diagnostic procedures other than the ones he has specifically requested; he will get truculent and loud when, instead of being rushed to the Operating Room, he is sent down to wait in X Ray for an abdominal film.

If the patient gets extremely disruptive and demanding, you can quickly quiet him down with a stern look and something along the lines

of "Tone it down, buster, or I won't operate at all!"

But be aware of the worst that can happen. The Medical Expert will not graciously accept it if, after your methodical workup involving lab tests and X Rays, damned if he doesn't have appendicitis after all! He will have a great big horse laugh at your expense.

The Holistic Patient; or, Suspicion Refractory to Usual Treatment

The Holistic Patient has many anxieties and fears about doctors, but is generally willing to talk about them. The hallmark of the Holistic Patient is a long list of questions brought to every appointment, which she reads off to you and takes notes:

- "Do you think of me as a case, a disease, or a whole person?"
- "Are there herbal/organic alternatives to this treatment?"
- "Aren't the pharmaceutical companies part of the right-wing military-industrial complex whose sole interest is in marketing and distributing unnecessary and useless placebos?"
- "Doesn't it strike you as bizarre that doctors make more money the sicker their patients are, rather than getting paid for keeping them well?"

You may be able, with patience, understanding, and many answers, to overcome the Holistic Patient's

The Medical Expert: Self-Diagnosis by the Average Joe

"Doc, you gotta operate!...
No, I don't want any X rays
or blood tests—just *operate*!"

The Holistic Patient

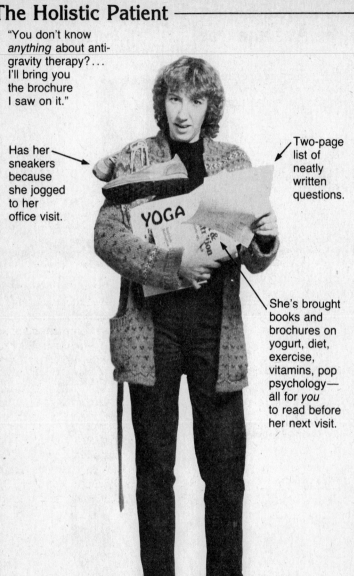

"You don't know *anything* about anti-gravity therapy?... I'll bring you the brochure I saw on it."

Has her sneakers because she jogged to her office visit.

Two-page list of neatly written questions.

YOGA

She's brought books and brochures on yogurt, diet, exercise, vitamins, pop psychology— all for *you* to read before her next visit.

deep distrust by establishing that you are not hateful, greedy, lazy, or ignorant. Unfortunately, it will take many years of intense questioning of your every decision, and many discussions of why penicillin really is a natural fungal product much like rose-hip tea before you reach that point in your doctor-patient relationship.

Sure-fire ways to completely alienate your Holistic Patient:

- "So when did *you* go to medical school?"
- "Yeah, I got news for you organic types—strychnine is a hundred percent natural, too!"
- "Oh, no! Not *another* article from that left-wing liberal rag, *Mother Jones*!"

The Stoic; or, "My wife made me come here, Doc"

The prototypical Stoic is a taciturn Maine farmer who last saw a doctor when he was born. He has come to see you only at the stubborn insistence of his wife, who is upset by the fact that he gets crushing chest pain and can't breathe every time he lifts firewood, calves, and bales of hay.

He is a straightforward fellow who wouldn't recognize a psychosomatic symptom if it came up and said, "Boo!" and doesn't even pay much mind to the little problems he's been having lately; it's only after much prodding by his wife that he will describe clear-cut symptoms of

a major disease. Doctors love this kind of patient, because he gives them an opportunity to treat a real disease in a solid citizen.

The Stoic will take his medicine regularly, he will call after office hours only if something is really wrong, he'll be grateful, and he'll pay his bills with a reasonable lag. Every fall, he'll send down a bushel of good apples from his farm in thanks.

The Drug-Seeker; or, "C'mon, just a quick pick-me-up, okay?"

Drug abusers cross every social and ethnic line. The Shaker Heights housewife swathed in Papagallo might be just as desperate for her Valium refill as the scuzzy denizen of the street or the high-school punk is for his Percodans.

Recreational, not medicinal, drugs are the issue when:

- *The patient asks for them by street name.* Be alerted when someone says, "What I really need for this terrible back pain are some Perks" (or some Roche 10's, T's and B's, Black Beauties, or Red Screamers).
- *The patient has three pieces of ID or more*, all with the same photo but different names.
- *The patient threatens bodily harm* when you suggest that aspirin might be a good idea.
- *The patient perks up when you say, "You seem to have some serious pain,"* but gets upset when you

continue, "so serious that I think we should admit you to the hospital and really figure out what is causing this pain, rather than just masking it with more narcotics."

- *The patient disappears while you are calling the police.*

The Doctor's Favorite Patient

Anyone, young or old, rich or poor, black or white, Republican or Democrat, with the attitude: "Doc, figure out what's wrong with me and fix it. I trust you. I know you'll do your best job. Do what you think is right."

Hallmark of the Favorite Patient: "Would you want your mother to have this operation? Okay, then, do it!"

The Stoic

"Crushing chest pain? Nah—Doc, I'm too much of a man to have pain!"

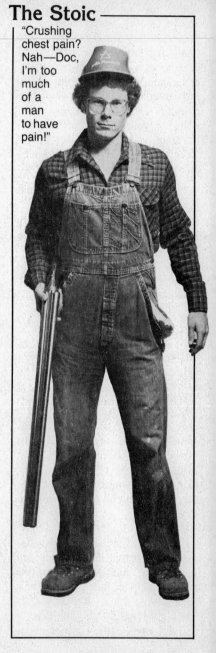

Customer Relations; or, Coping (Professionally) with Your Patients

Informed Consent: An Idea Whose Time Has Come (and Gone)

Legally and ethically, you, the doctor, must obtain "informed consent" from your patient before you perform any procedure on him. You must discuss the nature of the procedure, the reason you want to do it, what you will learn from it, the risks, the benefits, and the alternatives. Then the patient must sign a document certifying that you explained things to him.

In reality, however, most patients are so ill, anxious, and upset that they read a very different document from the one you put before them to sign.

THE ACTUAL INFORMED-CONSENT DOCUMENT

I, _____, understand and consent
to have the following procedure, _____,
performed on _____by _____
for the following reasons _____. The nature,
purpose, risks, and alternatives have been explained
to me. All my questions have been fully answered.

_____   _____
      Patient   Witness

                                 _____
                                           Witness

INFORMED CONSENT AS SEEN BY ADAM STOKES, COLLEGE PROFESSOR

I, _____, am signing away my life and limb to a man I've met once and instinctively dislike (recommended by my mother-in-law of all people!), whom I am allowing to perform an incredibly dangerous and probably unnecessary operation tomorrow so he can pay his kid's tuition at the Dalton School. Tomorrow he'll rummage around my guts, with a third-degree hangover or worse, and his mind only on his untrammeled lust for the operating-room nurse, and will probably cause more trouble than I've got already.

By signing this document I am no doubt waiving my legal right to sue him for all he's worth even if I wake up tomorrow a legless vegetable, but God forbid I should antagonize the man tonight by not signing his precious piece of paper when tomorrow a slip of his subconsciously hostile hand would mean The End!

_____   _____
    Lamb to Slaughter   Accomplices in Crime

                              _____

INFORMED CONSENT AS SEEN BY THE AVERAGE SICK PATIENT

Hey, do whatcha gotta do, Doc. Just fix me up and get me out of here.

_____   _____
        Patient   A Nurse

                              _____
                                  Another Nurse

INFORMED CONSENT AS SEEN BY THE SURGEON

I, _____, and my attorneys,
Squaliformes and Associates, are fully aware that
your scrap of paper means nothing in court—all I
have to say, is, "Yes, I read it, and signed it, but I
didn't *understand* it at the time." So kiss your 360
SEL good-bye should I end up with an icky scar, a
postoperative fever, a little malaise or depression, or,
God forbid, a sponge or clamp in my gut. Because we
will nail your rear fender to the wall!

           See you in court, sucker!

_____   Great White #1 _____

           Great White #2 _____

INFORMED CONSENT AS SEEN BY WILLIE KRETZKY,
BLUE-COLLAR WORKER

I, _____....What the hell? What is
this form, anyway? Is this the paper for signing away
my kidneys or something? Are things that bad? How
come no one told me? Where do I sign this thing? Or
does my wife sign it? Or both? Wish I had a beer
right now.

_____   _____

Is this where I sign it?   _____

                               Some ladies in the hall
                               who said they had to
                               sign it too. Maybe they
                               pick up the kidneys?

How to Avoid Getting Sued

Have you ever noticed that nurses' malpractice coverage costs about $100 a year while Orthopedic Surgeons pay more than $20,000 a year?

Do you know why this is?

Well, first, you can do more damage changing an artificial hip than you can do changing a bedpan.

Second, Orthopedic Surgeons make a lot more.

When people sue, they go for the deep pockets—and Orthopedic Surgeons have very deep pockets.

LOOK POOR. This is the key to avoiding lawsuits. Place a prominent sign in the parking lot that reads: DR. WATERHOUSE-FREDRICKSON'S PARKING SPACE, then buy a battered VW Bug and park it there day and night. Patients will think, first, that you keep incredibly long hours (and are therefore a virtuous person), and second, that you are far too poor to sue. After all, you're driving a car worse than their *teenager's* car! (Of course, *no one*

see you tooling home in the Jag you keep in the patients' parking lot.)

TALK POOR. An important corollary. Freely talk about your medical school and residency debts, your kids' college tuition debts, and your rotting roof and sinking swimming pool. (Don't bring up the incredible expense of country-club membership.)

ACT POOR. Be seen at cut-rate movie theaters still showing *E.T.* (you can always walk through and slip out the back). Be seen buying discount meats at the supermarket (no one needs to know that they're for your voracious Irish wolfhound). Talk about how terrible the subway system is (you don't actually have to *ride* on it).

What to Do if You (AAAUUGH!) Get Sued

You have three choices:

1. .357 Magnum to the temples— yours or the plaintiff's.

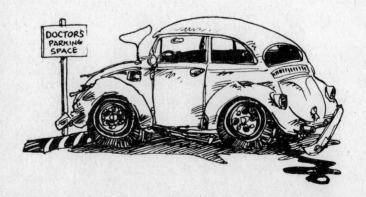

DOCTORS PARKING SPACE

2. Buy a one-way ticket to Caracas.
3. Hire a lawyer.

You may think that (3) is a logical choice. You would, of course, need a lawyer to represent you in court if you were being sued. But the medical opinion of the legal profession has long been less than complimentary, as can be seen from this story:

A doctor, a lawyer, and a priest were stranded on a desert isle surrounded by vicious, hungry sharks. The only means of escape was to swim through the shark-infested waters to a boat moored forty feet out.

"No way am I going to swim out there," said the doctor. "Besides, whoever does will need my immediate attention. So I can't do it."

"Well, I can't swim out there," said the priest, "because whoever does will need me, to administer last rites."

"Well," said the lawyer, "obviously my skills have no application in this situation. I'll do it!"

And with that he dived into the shark-infested waters and started swimming as hard and as fast as he could. All the sharks swam at him at breakneck speed—and then gently lifted him and carried him to the boat.

"I don't get it," said the doctor later, "Why'd they do that?"

"Oh," said the lawyer nonchalantly, "professional courtesy."

If you're getting sued, make sure you enlist the help of the best Great White possible to defend you—just don't go swimming with him!

No Bad Patients; The Woodhouse Way to Keep Your Patients in Line

You need to train your patients to do five things:

1. Take their medicine.
2. Keep their appointments.
3. Pay their bills.
4. Get better with your treatment.
5. *Never* think about lawsuits.

The Waiting Room as an Offensive Weapon

Waiting rooms are for waiting. Patients complain, but they secretly *like* to wait—it reinforces the idea that you are a busy, and therefore good, doctor.

To keep the 3 o'clocks waiting you may have to closet yourself in your office and watch *General Hospital* until 3:30. Just keep the sound down.

Keep the waiting room crowded. Encourage your receptionist's kids to do their homework in the waiting room. Have your wife do her knitting there. If you must, hire out-of-work actors to sit there and discuss in faintly British accents what an internationally famous doctor you are. All this may impress the one real patient you have sitting there.

Keep Your Patients Off Guard

Dress them in embarrassingly short, flimsy, open-backed gowns. These are useful both for optimal physical examination and for keeping your patient acutely uncomfortable. He will forget all of the incisive, critical questions he meant to ask in his efforts to get back into reasonable clothing. How seriously can you take a paunchy middle-aged man in one of those? More important, how seriously can he take himself?

Store all metallic equipment in a special refrigerator. At 40° F. Stethoscope, otoscope, and speculum should all be stored in there. And before seeing a patient, stick your hands in the fridge for a couple of minutes, too.

Decorate for Success: Creating an Intimidating Office

The combination of your forceful personality and your intimidating office atmosphere should so overwhelm the patient that he will cower in the low-set, uncomfortable patient's chair and say, "Yes, Doctor, whatever you think is right."

The forceful personality is up to you—be creative. But there are tried-and-true tips for office decor that are easy *and* effective.

Wallpaper the office with official-looking documents. Your M.D. and your residency certificates. Your Girl Scout Merit Badge for Needlework. Third Place in Junior Hunter at the Mamaroneck Horse Show. The warranty for your BMW. It makes absolutely no difference what you frame and tack to the wall—no one will ever read it. But everyone will be impressed.

Hang prints suitable to your specialty.

Psychiatrists: Munch's *The Scream* or Van Gogh's later, more psychotic paintings. Your patients will be reminded by these disconcerting paintings just how much they really need you.

Surgeons: Thomas Eakins' worshipful portraits of surgeons with halos behind their heads and their hands deep in bloody muck will inspire The Right Attitude in your patients—Awe and Fear.

Pediatricians: Any of the hopelessly idealized, Norman Rockwell-type portraits of childhood days, featuring adorable towheaded little boys getting into mischief, and kindly doctors giving shots to quietly weeping children. It hardly represents the chaos of your daily office, but it might lift the spirits of the bedraggled moms.

Obstetricians/Gynecologists: Anything by Mary Cassatt featuring beautiful slender mothers and rotund, healthy babies. (We all have our dreams and fantasies.)

Family Practitioners: No one expects a high-class operation from you. Hang admonitions from the

Public Health Department about smoking (the ones featuring Brooke Shields with cigarettes in her ears are quite popular); these will complement the reams of dusty, untouched Public Health brochures, on everything from birth control to weight loss, that sit in a listless pile year after untouched year.

Ophthalmologists: Optokinetic art from the late 1960s precipitates immediate and ineradicable headaches, and is difficult to clearly focus on. Or, of course, Magritte's *The False Mirror*.

Radiologists: No one ever goes down to the radiologists' office, which is generally a tiny cubicle in the rundown sub-basement of the hospital, so radiologists can freely express their eccentricities. Popular office decor includes charts of Egyptian hieroglyphics (to memorize between cases), lyrics from Gregorian chants (to recite while passing time), a retrospective of the year's centerfolds from the grimier skin magazines, or Crayola drawings (done while tripping).

The Common Medical Denominator: The Hippocratic Oath is a must for any doctor's office. Patients will be impressed by the lofty sentiment of the Oath, especially if it's set off by an elaborate gilt frame and a choice viewing location. A nice touch, even if you've never read the thing yourself.

Public Health Department Anti-Smoking Poster for Family Practitioner's Office

"I smoke for smell."

Be cool! DON'T smoke!

CHAPTER 15

How to Talk to Patients: A Primer of Bedside Manners

How to Explain Your Diagnosis and Treatment Plan

Utilize the vocabulary of your patients. For instance, your garage mechanic who needs coronary-by-pass surgery might best understand, "Your fuel line is clogged," whereas a business executive might better understand, "Decreased productivity in the last fiscal year by your heart indicates the need for a top-level replacement with a graft."

Don't oversimplify. Saying, "Well, dear, at your age things often go wrong 'down there'—you'll feel much perkier when that nasty womb is taken out," will get you written up in *Ms.* magazine's "No Comment" section, and you'll lose all your patients with I.Q.s higher than the inflation rate.

Don't get impatient. Especially, after your painstaking half-hour explanation of your diagnosis,

further tests, treatment, follow-up, and expectations for the course of the disease, when your patient says.

1. "Can you run all that by me again? I must've been day-dreaming."
2. "Can you call my wife in from the waiting room and explain all that to her?"
3. "Yo no hablo inglés."

Slip-sliding Away: How to Explain When You Don't have a Diagnosis

Explaining your diagnosis and treatment plan to a patient is child's play compared to explaining things when you have neither a diagnosis nor any clue as to what is wrong. Stay cool and calm. Remember the lessons you learned from those 6 A.M. Rounds when the Chief of Staff grilled you publicly on topics that you only vaguely understood. When in doubt, look confident. Radiate confidence. *Exude* confidence. Straighten your tie. Buff your shoes. Then face the music with your head held high. "Well, Mr. Jones, you have a set of puzzling symptoms. It isn't clear what exactly is wrong, although there are quite a few possibilities. However, we'll know more when we get the blood tests (or the brain biopsy or xerograms or T_3 resin uptake) back."

Important points to stress while giving this most unsatisfactory speech to your disappointed patient:

You, his doctor, will not sleep until you seek out and destroy his disease.

It is the complexity of his disease, NOT your inadequacy as a doctor, that prevents you from making a snap diagnosis.

Medicine is an Art, not a Science. You may *never* diagnose him. But that's not *your* fault; it's simply the trials and tribulations that accompany the artistic endeavor.

Hang crepe. Prepare the patient for the worst without scaring him to death; paint as grim a picture as possible without actually precipitating a double-gainer off the Golden Gate. Then, if everything goes well (and it turns out to be an old TB scar and not lung cancer), you can attribute it to your brilliant surgical skill or diagnostic acumen: "Well, Mrs. Trendelenberg, things were tight there for a while, but my incredible surgical ability pulled your

daughter through the worst of her nose job. I think she'll make it."

If everything goes wrong? Well, at least you accurately predicted it.

Don't let the patient overhear your comments to the office nurse. Hearing the doctor say, "I have no idea what's wrong with that guy, I wish I hadn't slept through my entire Endocrinology rotation. Look— check off every test Blue Cross will cover and schedule the guy back for an appointment. Maybe something will turn up," will NOT build patient confidence.

Pre-operative Conversation No-nos; or, What NOT to Say to Your Patients Before They Go into Surgery

- "Damn! I forgot my glasses! Have to operate without 'em, I guess."
- "Did I ever tie one on last night! I'm *still* seeing double—and just look at my hands shake. Better lay off the coffee."
- "Well, I hope this one turns out better than the last patient I did; he bought the farm last night."
- "Sometimes I get so depressed. I never should have gone into surgery. It's hard to face, but I'm just not that good at it!"

Intra-operative Conversation No-nos; or, Remember That Local Anesthesia Does NOT Affect Patient's Hearing

1. "Oops!" (Or any variant thereof.)
2. "Oh, c'mon, let the Medical Student try—she's got to learn *sometime.*"
3. "Oh, Jesus. *Now* what are we going to do?"
4. "What's *that? Bowel?* Aren't we a bit, uh, *deep?*"

How to Break Good News About a Diagnosis

1. Take credit for it.
2. Stress how important it was to have the procedure done, even though it was painful, unpleasant, expensive, and came back negative. "Now I know it was icky to lie on a sigmoidoscope table for forty-five minutes while the GI doctor tried to snag that little polyp through an eighteen-inch steel tube up your rectum, but it's important we know everything's okay."
3. Share in the experience; stress how relieved you both are. "Now we can both sleep at night, free from anxieties about those worrisome symptoms."

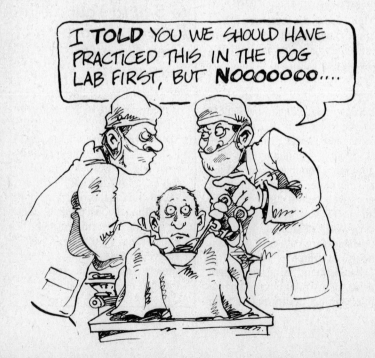

I **TOLD** YOU WE SHOULD HAVE PRACTICED THIS IN THE DOG LAB FIRST, BUT **NOOOOOOO**....

4. Ascertain that the patient really wants to hear the good news. A surprising number of otherwise reasonable people, brainwashed by Ali MacGraw's demise from leukemia, think that leukemia would be a dramatic and beautiful way to go (unaware as they are that leukemics do *not* die with prefectly teased hairdos, Bermuda suntans, and rosy cheeks by Revlon, but rather with mouth ulcerations, perirectal abscesses, wall-to-wall bruises, and whole-body pain). These people are quite disappointed to hear that they've got mononucleosis, not leukemia, and that they have to go *right back* to junior high in one week.

Other people leverage illnesses to avoid unpleasant situations or duties ("Not tonight, dear, I might have a brain tumor"), or use their "illnesses" as an excuse for failure ("My doctor thinks there might be something wrong with my thyroid. I just can't lose weight, no matter how hard I try, so I might as well have another piece of cheesecake... with strawberries").

Don't be surprised when these patients take the good news with poor grace. It isn't that they don't believe you ("Doc! You must be wrong! I feel like I'm gonna die")—it's just that they're thinking of all the garbage they'll have to carry out now that they don't have heart disease, and all the guff they're going to get from people who have regarded them as hypochondriacs and shirkers for years and now have proof.

You must adopt a strongly positive sales technique to absolutely prove to these people that 1) their protoplasm is healthy and hale, and 2) they should be happy about this. It helps to have tangible proof like X rays and biopsies on hand.

Not just: "See? Your coronary angiogram is normal."

But instead: "Look how *wide* these coronary arteries are, and how smooth! These nice healthy blood vessels let all the strong oxygenated blood through, like a flood of New York marathoners rushing across the Brooklyn Bridge."

The Lighter Side of Terminal Illness: How to Break Bad News

People take death, especially their own, quite seriously. They won't be in the mood for your best Groucho Marx routine, no matter how well it went over at the last staff meeting.

There are many ways to reveal a diagnosis. The following will certainly make things more interesting for you (although they may disconcert your patients).

• "I've got some good news and some bad news. The good news is we have a diagnosis. The bad news is it's cancer."

• "The good news is there's a treatment for this cancer. The bad news is that it will increase your life expectancy from only three to nine months."

• "Let me put it this way: Don't buy any long-playing records."

• "You know how you really hate winter in Boston? Well, next year you won't have to put up with it! You won't *be* here!"

But seriously, there are a few guidelines that, if observed, will make your job easier:

• *Break bad news to the correct family*. When you emerge from an unsuccessful eight-hour marathon attempt to surgically save William Dohle-Heller after he blew out a syphilitic aortic sinusal aneurysm and lost enough blood to stock the Minneapolis blood bank for a week), make damned sure that you tell Mr. Dohle-Heller's family, and not the Palatine family, who is waiting to hear how little Jimmy Palatine's tonsillectomy went (unless precipitating mass hysteria is your idea of a fun time).

• *Make sure the family is sitting before you let loose with the big black headlines*. Six large Italian matrons simultaneously fainting creates quite a ruckus, and blocks the food carts, too.

• *Let the patient in on the news first*. Twenty-seven teary relatives descending on him, smothering him with weepy kisses, begging forgiveness for past transgressions, and

dropping heavy-handed hints about his will, might indicate to the patient that perhaps, just possibly, all is not well.

• *Look on the bright side*. This is especially important for Obstetricians, who are frequently involved in touchy doctor-patient situations. An Obstetrician delivering a hermaphrodite might try, "Congratulations! It's an it!" or "You know how you were undecided whether you wanted a boy or a girl? Well, you've got both!" Of course, not all deliveries are so complicated; hermaphrodites are few and far between, while merely ugly babies are born everyday. One well-intentioned Obstetrician tried to console the mother after the birth of a particularly ugly baby by saying, "Well, it's indisputable that you've got a really ugly-looking kid there, Mrs. Braxton-Hicks, but look at it this way: beauty isn't everything. Why, look how far *you've* come in life!" (This particular Obstetrician escaped serious bodily harm only because he had the aforementioned Mrs. Braxton-Hicks firmly strapped in stirrups.)

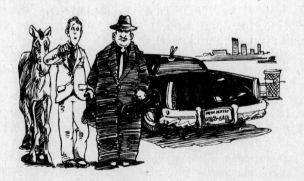

CHAPTER 16

Families and Friends of Your Patients: Wild in the Streets (and in Your Nice Clean Hospital Corridors)

Moments of crisis are not the only times that you will have to interface with your patients' friends and families; these loved ones will inevitably be underfoot for the duration of every patient's hospital stay. It's enough to drive the calmest M.D. wild! But remember your goal (to cure your patients), and always keep in mind whom you're dealing with, and you'll be fine.

Certain patients' families should be treated with utmost respect and caution. Arnold Chiari's brother Bud, for instance. The guy who drives a stretch limo with Jersey plates, wears dark blue sharkskin suit, and doesn't laugh at Secretary of Labor Donovan jokes. Don't get on Bud Chiari's bad side—a little slip of the scalpel and both you and your daughter's pony will be in hot water.

Respect ethnic rituals of sickness. Draw the line, though, at practices that upset the nurses: goats and chickens, for instance, are out, and a ritual slaughter of a spring lamb for good luck will make a lot of extra work for Housekeeping.

Fun Things That Visitors Bring to Patients

- *cookies, candy, and cake for the teenage diabetic* ("Just a secret treat—don't tell those fussy doctors!")
- *quick pick-me-up shots of heroin* into the convenient intravenous line from well-wishing fellow addicts
- *hair-raising medical exposés* from newspapers like *The National En-*

153

quirer for the post-operative patient:

"Fifty-Seven Drugs That Can Cripple or Kill you"

"Avoid Painful and Unnecessary Surgery from Greedy Surgeons"

"Most American Doctors Are Schizophrenic and I Can Prove It"

And the all-time classic: *"Your Doctor: Enemy or Foe?"*

Charming Things That Visitors Say to Patients

It is a bit of a shock to see someone in the hospital. Put Christopher Reeves into a hospital bed wearing an ugly short gown, deprive him of a shave, shower, sunlight, and barbells for a few days, plug in a few intravenous lines and a nasogastric suction tube, feed him hospital food, and even superman will look like a sick basset hound.

This debilitated state of being automatically deprives the visitor of the optimal opening gambit— "Chris! You old shyster! You look terrific"—and instead shocks him into blurting out, "You poor kid! You look like death warmed over!"

This will not cheer your patient.

Other favorite topics visitors choose:

Particulars of domestic turmoil:

1) loss of income because of illness
2) kids failing out of school
3) roof of house falling in
4) ex-husband stopped by to gloat.

Hot office gossip

1) how well the office is doing without the patient
2) what a terrific job the patient's temporary replacement is doing
3) more RIFs and forced retirements are looming
4) prospective top-level management shake-up, including the patient's job.

Terrifying descriptions of other friends' and relatives' surgical complications:

1) Aunt Bertha, who was fit as a fiddle but dropped dead right after having the same operation the patient had
2) people who never woke up from anesthesia
3) obstetrical disaster stories—especially to first-time, extremely anxious expectant mothers— about dead babies and brain-injured mothers.

But always remember who you are: you are the Doctor. Your word is Law—at least in the hospital— and your primary responsibility is to your patient. If your patient *wants* the entire extended family to wail twenty-four hours a day by his bedside, reinforcing their dedication to him as he contemplates another rewrite of his will, fine. Maybe the old codger enjoys the attention. But if the domestic hysteria is wearing him down, exercise your medical authority and send them all home— it will do you both some good.

CHAPTER 17

Doctorspeak; or, Why Dyspareunia is Better Than No Pareunia at All

Make up your own medical words! Doctors love to use obscure medical jargon instead of everyday lay language; rather than say "slow heart rate," they will say *bradycardia* (*brady* = slow, *cardia* = heart), and painful sex sounds much more official as *dyspareunia* (*dys* = painful, *pareunia* = sex). Patients, too, seem to find it comforting that actual medical terms exist for their problems, and doctors like to use medical labels to justify their huge itemized bills.

But doctorspeak is not limited to the experienced members of the medical world and their patients alone; with practice, anyone can authoritatively fling about medical jargon, and even create an entire vocabulary. Just use the handy prefixes, suffixes, and roots listed below. For example, just had your heart broken in a disastrous love affair? You need a *cardiopexy!* (*cardio* = heart, *pexy* = to fix). How do

you describe surgery when the surgeon is very slow? *Bradyectomy* (*brady* = slow, *ectomy* = surgical removal). And what do you call a highly paid subspecialist who is raking in the megabucks at top speed? A *tachymonetriatrist,* of course, (*tachy* = fast, *monetri* = money, *iatrist* = specialist). Even patients get a kick out of adopting bits and pieces of doctorspeak for their own uses; depending on your patient population, you may hear patients respond to pain with such original phrases as "brady lordy" or "tachy oy."

Abbreviations

Doctors love abbreviations; in fact, they can frequently be heard conversing in sustained sentences comprised entirely of abbreviations, with only a few stray verbs to cement them together. For example, there is documented proof that the

Prefixes

an = without	infra = below	pre = before
ante = before	intra = within	retro = behind
brady = slow	mal = disordered	sub = under
dia = between	meta = changing	supra = over
hypo = below	post = after	tachy = fast

Roots

adeno = gland	chole = gall	derma = skin	hemo = blood
arthro = joint	cranio = skull	entero = intestine	hepato = liver
cardi = heart	cysto = bladder	gastro = stomach	hystero = uterus

Suffixes

algia = pain	itis = inflammation	ostomy = creating an opening
desis = fusion	lysis = freeing of	pathy = abnormality
dynia = pain	oma = tumor	pexy = fix in place
ectomy = surgical removal		plasty = restore or reconnect
iatrist = specialist	oscopy = viewing	rrhea = flow or discharge

following sentence was uttered yesterday at a major teaching hospital:

> The Dx was COPD and we R/ Out MI or a PE; we d/c'd the I.V. and he's not N.P.O. We're just waiting for the CT and V̇/Q̇ now.*

Abbreviations don't always mean what they sound like: SOB is *shortness of breath*, not a pain-in-the-neck patient. RN stands for *Really Nasty*, although nurses would like you to believe it stands for *registered nurse*.

*The *diagnosis* was *chronic obstructive pulmonary disease* and we *ruled out myocardial infarction* or *pulmonary embolus;* we *discontinued* the *intravenous* and he's not *nothing by mouth* (latin: *per os*); we're just waiting for the *computerized axial tomography* and *ventilation/perfusion scan* now.

(*LPN*, the title for the RN's less-trained counterpart, stands for *large pain in neck*.) And a medical *T and A* is nowhere near as exciting as its show-biz counterpart—somehow a *tonsillectomy and adenoidectomy* sounds a lot less intriguing than *tits and ass*. Unless, of course, you're in ENT (Ears, Nose, and Throat).

The ABCs of Doctorspeak: A Glossary

A is for Attending: The staff physician in an academic institution who supervises residents' patient care. The Attending expounds at will on American Medicine Today to his captive audience of Medical Students and Residents, whose future careers depend on his favor; favorite theme is "Back when I was a Resident, and men were men...and Residents were poorly paid, worked harder, and complained less." Generally this speech is given to Residents who have worked the last thirty-six hours without sleep. *Identifying Feature of the Attending:* Stays awake on Rounds; only member of the team to do so.

A is also for Arrest: Cardiac Arrest is the great social event of any hospital night. You run like hell through the hospital corridors To Save A Life (the most dramatic minutes of your medical career, with a full audience of awed visitors and patients) and arrive at a room to find either (if you are too early) a tubercular gomer who has aspirated his vomitus and had a respiratory and cardiac arrest, on whom you are obligated to initiate mouth-to-mouth resuscitation until your team arrives, or (if you are too late) a room full of milling Residents with four people actively engaged in pumping the chest, checking the blood pressure, watching the EKG, pumping the Ambu bag, and administering drugs. (As you can see, arriving too late isn't bad at all—it's a great opportunity to catch up on hospital gossip, see who's in house, and get free consults—all without having to do any real work. Any way you look at it, arriving last at a code is better than arriving first and picking up God knows what Killer Bee bacteria.

B is for Boxed: A.K.A. Bought the Farm, Kicked the Bucket, A Situation Incompatible with Life—all terms for what you do not want your patient to do.

C is for Crump: Crumping is what the patient does shortly before he boxes. Also referred to as circling the drain, crashing, or having one foot on a banana peel, the other in the grave. It is a general rule that patients crump when:
1. It is between 2 and 5 A.M.
2. The intern is swamped with admissions.
3. The Intensive Care Unit nurses are on strike.

D is for Debt: That which you are deeply in.

D is also for Delta: "No delta" means no change; is seen frequently in the cryptic surgeons' progress notes as "Patient O.K. No Δ."

E is for Emergency Medical Center: also known as
1 Doc-in-the-Box
2 McDocs
3 Mediquick/Mediquack

E is also for Euboxic: Eu is the Latin root for "true"; box refers to the little boxed charts that lab results come on. Euboxic means all the lab numbers fit in the boxes, and the patient's labs are normal. Also known as "Harvard numbers."

F is for FMG: Foreign Medical Graduate, a dubious distinction. The mention of the Autonomous Universidad de Guadalajara is always good for a laugh at a doctors' cocktail party.

G is for Gomer: Any patient who has been frozen in a comatose fetal position since the Truman administration, has seventeen volumes in his medical chart, and whose last verbal communication was "Bess, is that you?" in the spring of 1968 and who since then has only said "GAAAH" every fifteen minutes for fifteen years. Derived either from the acronym "*G*et *O*ut of *M*y *E*mergency *R*oom" or from Gomer Pyle.

H is for House: House in medical jargon is not your *home*, but the hospital. Therefore, patients are admitted *to* the house, and residents are trapped *in* the house.

H is also for Hit: Verb or noun, meaning a patient whom a Resident must admit, usually two to three hours of nocturnal work. *Example* "Six hits and it's only 2 A.M.! I'm not going to sleep tonight!"

I is for Indignity: No hospital experience is complete without indignities—ranging from the petty, like "How are we today, Betty?" from a nurse young enough to be your great-granddaughter, to the gross indignities that are better left unspecified.

I is also for "I's & O's": the abbreviation for *Intake & Output*, the record of a patients' fluid balance. One med student, told to check a patient's I's & O's, came back and said, "His eyes and nose look fine to me."

J is for Jumping Ship: What every Medical Student is tempted to do at some juncture in his/her career.

K is for Potassium: "What's his $K+$?" is the standard Cardiologist's question. It's okay not to really *understand* the significance of electrolyte levels, but woe to the Medical Student or Resident who doesn't at least know the numbers.

L is for Leisure Time: Not in your vocabulary.

M is for Medical Student: S/He who can do no right.

Most Frequent Statement:
"I'm probably wrong, but..."
Most Frequent Activity: Doing
Something Wrong.
Identifying Characteristic:
Hopelessly confused.

N is for Nurse:
1. Someone who can help you, and doesn't.
2. Someone who can hurt you, and does.

N is also for No-Code: A patient who has been designated not to be resuscitated if she arrests on the basis of
1. Intractable terminal disease.
2. Family wishes.
3. Objectionable personality that bugs the Residents.

O is for O Sign: The *O Sign* is the International Sign of the Gomer, a toothless unresponsive patient who lies with his mouth open all day.

P is for The Pit: The Emergency Room, where all Residents must go down to pick up new admissions, is The Pit. Getting stuck in The Pit all night is a fate commensurate with, if not actually worse than, death.

Q is for The Q Sign: Corollary to the *O Sign*. A patient with his mouth open and tongue hanging out. The *Dotted Q Sign* is when a fly lands on the tongue.

R is for Resident: An M.D. engaged in postgraduate training for three to nine years, at wages less than the average postman earns.
Synonymous with: scutbunny, pumpboy, slave, "hey boy!"
Most frequent activities: Sleeping standing up, getting dumped on by Attendings, berating Students, making unreasonable demands on nurses, going through messy divorces.
Most common phrase: "Honey, I can't get home tonight—why do you think they call us *Residents?*"

R is also for Rounds: A sophisticated form of torture directed at Medical Students and lower-level Residents; ostensibly a didactic session in which cases are discussed, but actually designed to accentuate each Resident's or Medical Student's ignorance, sloth, and lack of moral character.

S is not for Sleep: Not in your vocabulary.

S is for STAT: the order to do something very quickly. In most hospitals STAT or ASAP means someone will get around to it after coffee break, or maybe next week.

S is also for Spouse: The girl/boy you left behind.
Most frequent phrase: "If I wanted to spend all my time

alone, I *wouldn't* have gotten married!"

Identifying feature: You don't remember.

Favorite activity: Suing for divorce on grounds of neglect.

T is for Turf: Alert Residents find reasons to transfer or "turf" their patients to other services, which results in less work. Medicine service patients who fracture a hip can be "turfed" to Orthopedics. Orthopedics patients with pneumonia can be "turfed" to medicine. Vets can be "turfed" to the V.A.

T is also for "Therapeutic Adventure": Clinical disaster when everything that can go wrong—confused medicines, wrong operation, power failure—does.

U is for Unit: The Intensive Care Unit, where patients are sent when they crash. Also where the Intern gets to stay up all night keeping the crashing patient from boxing.

V is for Veterans Administration Hospitals: V.A.s (affectionately known as *V.A. Spas*), are training grounds for millions of American doctors. Generally the pits to work in, with none of the charm of suburban hospitals. Surviving a V.A. is similar to living through a fraternity hazing.

W is for Wall: Noun; greatly admiring term for Resident manning the Emergency Room who doesn't admit patients but instead treats and releases them. The derisive term, for the resident who admits anybody complaining of headache, is a Sieve, as in "There's a sieve in the E.R.—we'll be awake all night!"

W is also for WNL: Most common abbreviation, seen on medical charts all over the country. Stands for "Within Normal Limits," in reference to the physical examination of a body part, although most doctors maintain that it really stands for "We Never Looked."

X- is for X-ray doctors: Radiologists, also known as The Shadow Doctors.

Y is for Yawn: What you are unable to suppress throughout the day.

Z is for Zebra: The rarest of rare diseases. Medical Students like to make bizarre and unusual diagnoses, such as "quasireliculated hairy-cell dysgerminoma" instead of a simple wart, "Tutsugamushi fever" instead of the flu. A frequent admonition to them is "When you hear hoofbeats, look for horses, not zebras."

Why It's Better to Be a Doctor than a Patient

1. There's a good chance you'll leave the hospital alive.
2. You wear a nifty white coat, not a ridiculous little gown.
3. You *chose* to be in the hospital, and you get *paid* for being there.
4. You can go out for lunch. And home for dinner. *Maybe*.
5. It hurts a lot less to do an appendectomy than to have one done.
6. You can boss the nurses around, not vice versa.
7. You're one of the few people who can actually give *Informed* Consent (not that you ever would).

Why It's Better to Be a Patient than a Doctor

1. It isn't.

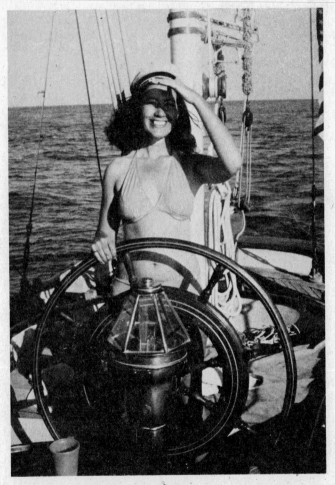

Anne Eva Ricks, M.D., an Alpha Omega Alpha graduate of the University of Cincinnati, wants to be the doctor on *The Love Boat* when she grows up.